The Ship Captain's Medical Guide

Harry Leach

THE SHIP CAPTAIN'S

MEDICAL GUIDE.

LONDON: PRINTED BY
SPOTTISWOODE AND CO., NEW-STREET SQUARE
AND PARLIAMENT STREET

OFFICIAL NOTICE.

———◆———

The Board of Trade have sanctioned this Book in the following words :—

WHEREAS it is provided by the 'Merchant Shipping Act, 1867,' as follows, viz.:—

The Board of Trade shall from time to time issue and cause to be published Scales of Medicines and Medical Stores suitable for different ships and voyages, and shall also prepare or sanction a book or books containing instructions for dispensing the same :

The owners of every ship navigating between the United Kingdom and any place out of the same shall provide and cause to be kept on board such ship a supply of medicines and medical stores in accordance with the scale appropriate to the said ship, and also a copy of the said book, or of one of the said books, containing instructions :

Now THEREFORE, in pursuance of the powers vested in them by provisions above recited, the Board of Trade hereby sanction a Book of Instructions, for dispensing the medicines and medical stores provided and kept on board ship, intituled 'The Ship Captain's Medical Guide,' price One Shilling and Threepence, compiled by HARRY LEACH, resident Medical Officer of the 'Dreadnought' Hospital Ship, and Inspector of lime and lemon juice appointed by the Board of Trade for the Port of London.

Given under the Seal of the Board of Trade, this 14th day of September 1868.

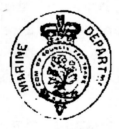

THOMAS GRAY,
*One of the Assistant Secretaries
to the said Board.*

THE SHIP CAPTAIN'S

MEDICAL GUIDE.

COMPILED BY

HARRY LEACH,

RESIDENT MEDICAL OFFICER HOSPITAL-SHIP '.DREADNOUGHT

SECOND EDITION.

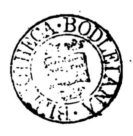

LONDON:
SIMPKIN, MARSHALL, AND CO.

STATIONERS'-HALL COURT.

1868.

Price One Shilling and Threepence.

PREFACE.

THIS WORK is written solely for the use of Masters and Mates of vessels at sea. It is confined strictly to a plain and brief description of accidents and diseases that occur on board ship; and much care has been taken to show, as clearly as possible, how these accidents and diseases can be best treated by a non-professional man. So little choice is given in the treatment of each malady, that the reader is urged to do absolutely all that is recommended, in the belief that no more than is here laid down can be accomplished safely without the assistance of a doctor. The chapters that treat of accidents and surgical diseases are, for the most part, the work of Dr. H. T. L. Rooke, Surgeon to the 'Dreadnought' Hospital Ship; and Dr. W. Dickson, R.N., Medical Inspector of Her Majesty's Customs, has given most valuable assistance in the work of revision. The compiler begs to offer many acknowledgments for the aid that has been so courteously afforded to him, and commends this book to the earnest attention of Commanders in the Mercantile Marine, hoping to receive from their experience suggestions that may tend to its completeness and consolidation.

CONTENTS.

———◦◦◦———

ACCIDENTS.

POISONS.

MEDICAL DISEASES.

THE

SHIP CAPTAIN'S MEDICAL GUIDE.

—◦◦—

GENERAL REMARKS.

ALL READERS of this book will be agreed that the
interests of owners as well as commanders of ships
are most powerfully aided by sending every vessel to
sea with a sound and healthy crew.   Art has accomplished a great deal in diminishing the gross amount
of manual labour now required on board ship, and
patent reefing topsails, improved running gear, and
many other recent changes have done much in assist-
ing to reduce the number of hands required to ensure all proper speed, and all possible precautionary
means of safety.   But, as no vessel can ever be
entirely independent of her crew, it is eminently
necessary that she should haul out of dock with a
robust supply (as to quality) of hands ; that, as far as
is possible, the good men shall not be called upon
to do the work of the sickly as well as their own ;

B

and that all on the articles shall have a chance of 'starting fair.'

It is believed that the 10th section of The Merchant Shipping Act (extracts from which may be found at the end of this book) might, if faithfully carried out, do much to effect this very desirable object. All captains know to their cost the excessive inconvenience and serious losses that arise from shipping unhealthy men for a long voyage; men who, as soon as the ship has put to sea, present themselves aft with a bad rupture, a large ulcer, a big bubo, or a diseased heart, lay up for days, weeks, and months, give thereby additional labour to the rest of the watch, and eventually take money from the owners that they have in no wise earned. The adoption of this section of the act will give a practical surety to the captain that his crew are in as good order as his spars and gear, to the crew that they will not be compelled to do more than a fair day's work for a fair day's wage, and to the owner that he will really get a fair day's work out of every hand shipped.

It is now a duty to tell the reader that the following pages are written with the object of showing not only what to *do* in cases of accident and sickness, but what to *avoid*. Doctors have lately learnt much on this head, and will tell you that in the practice of their own profession much harm may be done to the body by meddling and muddling. It is very important that this fact should be widely known, and so, acting thereupon, let the reader remember and apply the following rules:—

(1) Follow out strictly all the recommendations enjoined in this book.

(2) Do not take with you or use any medicines other than those inserted in the official scale.

(3) When in doubt as to the nature of a disease, wait and watch.

Struggle hard and actively to *prevent* disease, but when you are called upon to *cure*, adopt the directions given here, meagre as they may appear, and believe (as you may most assuredly do) that your own humble efforts to restore health and prolong life will receive safe and splendid backing from the wonderful hand of Nature.

PREVENTION OF DISEASE.

MANY DISEASES are much more easily prevented than cured.

This is a fact that cannot be too forcibly impressed upon the minds of men who have the sole and entire charge of any community of human beings, ashore or afloat. The professional knowledge acquired by a doctor now very largely includes the art of prevention, and commanders of ships may be assured that this art can be acquired, in a great degree, by all who will take the trouble to observe how much the health of the body depends upon proper food, pure air, cleanliness of skin, and garments suited to the weather.

Keep the sleeping-places clean, dry, and well ventilated. Let the men have dry and warm clothing, and an occasional change of diet, with vegetables and other antiscorbutics. Exercise judgment and discretion in dealing with your crew, and you will do much to remove the chances of disease.

Your forecastle, deckhouse, cabins, and galley should be thoroughly cleaned out, washed and swabbed down, once a week. The hold should be cleaned in the same way as often as is possible, and carbolic acid (see page 69) should be used in the process. A small quantity of this acid given to the boatswain will last, for this purpose, two or three months, and will sweeten the men's quarters in a very great degree. Do not use more acid in the water than is directed (on page 69), or you will injure the wood, iron, and gear of the ship.

If any contagious disease has broken out, sprinkle this mixture of water and carbolic acid over the quarters and berths every day, and give your men an opportunity of using it for washing purposes, according to the directions given.

Keep patients suffering from contagious diseases as far as possible from the rest of the crew.

SCURVY.—Until very great changes are made, by mutual agreement on the part of owners and seamen, in the scales of diet now commonly used in long-voyage ships, this disease must be *prevented* by constant care in the giving out of limejuice.

The operation of The Merchant Shipping Act, 1867 (extracts from which may be found at the end of this book) will ensure to all ships a genuine and palatable supply of this article. The juice will contain sufficient rum or other spirit to give it a ' groggy ' flavour. All vessels proceeding east of the Cape of Good Hope and west of Cape Horn should be furnished with a supply sufficient for at least twelve months', and vessels to all other ports with a supply sufficient for eight months' consumption, according to the number of hands on board. Make your steward mix it according to the following scale, and serve it out to each man at dinner every day:—

	Limejuice	Water	Sugar
For 10 men . .	½ pt. (10 oz.)	6 pts.	10 oz.
„ 15 „ . .	¾ pt. (15 oz.)	9 pts.	15 oz.
„ 20 „ . .	1 pt. (20 oz.)	12 pts.	20 oz.

More water may be added if preferred by the men.

It is believed that all hands will gladly take this mixture. You will understand that no limejuice can be legally used on board ship unless it is certified by an Inspector, and obtained from a Customs' Bonded Warehouse. You and your owners are responsible that a sufficient quantity is shipped; *you* are responsible that it is mixed properly, and served out regularly day by day. If you do not serve it out, or see it served out, and the men become ill in consequence, you will be liable for the consequences of such illness, and also to a penalty. If any of your crew neglect to drink it, they do so at their own peril, and you are bound to record every such neglect in the Official Log-book of the ship (see page 80).

Give a double allowance to any man who has spots on his skin from venereal disease.

CHOLERA.—You may prevent this disease by persuading your men to come aft directly looseness of the bowels commences, and then by treating them as directed in this book (see page 45).

RHEUMATISM.—This malady may, in most cases, be prevented by dry berths and dry warm clothing. It is far safer to sweat from heat than to shiver from cold, whether in cold, temperate, or tropical latitudes.

AGUE (or the fever, as it is commonly called).— You may prevent this disease by giving your men four grains of quinine every morning when they turn out. Recollect this very useful precaution on the west coast of Africa, in the West Indies, about the north-east coast of South America, in China, and the East India islands.

VENEREAL DISEASES.—These maladies have always been the bane of the mercantile marine service, and the indirect causes of loss of life and property to an extent that few persons have as yet realised. A captain may start from any home or foreign port, may soon discover a condition of things briefly described on page 2, and at a time when scarcity of hands indicates imminent risk to the ship and to all on board. The 10th section of the Merchant Shipping Act, 1867 (see page 82), was passed for the purpose of giving the owners and masters of ships an opportunity of ascertaining, as far as possible, whether seamen applying for employment are labouring under any disease likely to incapacitate them for sea service. If you do not avail yourself of the opportunities for medical examination of your crew placed at your disposal by that Act, you should at least do what you can to reduce the chances of the crew becoming demoralised and debauched whilst they are under your orders, and especially to *prevent* venereal diseases among your crews whilst the vessel is in port abroad. Much may be done by an active mate in making the ship comfortable, so that, when the work of discharging or taking in cargo is over for the day, the excessive anxiety for shore-leave will be less marked. Give your men the opportunity of obtaining good tobacco, and, if possible, good beer or other liquor on board, as well as any other extras that they may wish to buy; and, at ports where newspapers are published or sold, let them have copies without stint. Make the hour of shore-leave as early as possible, and encourage the men to apply to the doctor that you employ, directly after the occurrence of any symptoms of venereal disease, by reminding them that neglect on this head may lead to a forfeiture of their wages, according to the 8th sec. of The Merchant Shipping Act, 1867 (see page 82). Above all things it should be understood that personal cleanliness is one of the best means of prevention.

DRUNKENNESS.—The means adopted for the prevention of venereal diseases in foreign ports will apply with equal force to the vice of drunkenness. The bad quality, fully as much as the large quantity, of drink swallowed by sailors, is a fruitful source of liver diseases, dysentery, and other ills. Do all that you can to lesson the inducements to frequent those villainous haunts where poisonous drinks and foul women speedily make your men utterly useless and burdensome to you and to themselves.

DYSENTERY.—This disease (see page 46) affects most severely the crews of ships lying at Calcutta, Hong-Kong, Bombay, Kurrachee, and Foo-Chow-Foo, and there is no doubt that its prevalence at these ports is due to the bad quality of the water used for drinking purposes. It is therefore your duty and interest to prevent or mitigate this miserable and often fatal malady, by making great efforts to obtain a good water supply when in port, and also for the homeward passage. Much of the scurvy brought from Calcutta is attributed by captains and mates to the badness of the water, but the experience of doctors goes to prove that dysentery, rather than scurvy, follows the use of bad water. It is, however, sometimes impossible to obtain a supply of good water; and if your ship is not provided with a distilling apparatus, it will be advisable to obtain, before leaving port, two or three large filters. These valuable articles are now so commonly used, and are so very cheap, that the trouble and cost of carriage are amply repaid by the aid they will afford in the prevention of disease. Filters may be obtained in England for use on board ship at a cost, according to size, of from fifteen shillings to three or four pounds each. They will purify from six to seventy-two gallons of water per day. If you have no filters, all suspected water should be purified by adding two or three drops of Condy's Fluid (which will be found in the medicine chest) to each gallon of water.

Much illness of various kinds will be prevented by seeing that your men are exposed to the influence of rain and tropical sun as little as possible, and that a fair time is always allowed for meals, and for the maintenance of proper cleanliness both as to body and berths.

ACCIDENTS.

NOTE.—When bandages are necessary, they should be put on very smoothly and evenly, with moderate pressure, and should be kept very clean. Dirty dressings do more harm than good.

WOUNDS.

WOUNDS may be clean-cut, ragged, pierced, poisoned, or caused by a gun-shot.

CLEAN-CUT WOUNDS, made by a sharp instrument, if not very deep or long, are not dangerous, though they may bleed freely.

Treatment.—Cleanse the wound from dirt, bring the cut edges close to each other and keep them together by strapping, or by a fine needle and thread passed through the sides, and tied in a reef knot; over the cut surface place a pad of lint, and fix it with strapping.

RAGGED WOUNDS.—In these cases the flesh is more or less torn, and the edges are jagged and unequal.

Treatment.—There is but little bleeding, and the edges being ragged and bruised, it is useless to bring them closely together. Apply lint dipped in cold water or in the carbolic acid lotion (see page 76), and if the pain be great, warm fomentations or poultices. When the inflammation has subsided, warm-water dressing soonest heals the wound.

PIERCED WOUNDS OR STABS.—These are much more dangerous than clean cuts, on account of their depth. Vital parts may be injured, the point of the weapon may break off, and be left in the wound, and these wounds are very likely to be followed by inflammation, fever, and deep abscesses.

Treatment.—At first, lint dipped in cold water should be applied and kept constantly wet. With this simple treatment the wound will occasionally heal. If, however, it throbs, and is hot and painful, matter is about to form. Hot poultices should then be applied, and changed frequently. If the patient be feverish, he must have a free purge, and then take the fever mixture three times a day (page 74).

POISONED WOUNDS.—The most simple are those caused by stings of bees, wasps, hornets, and other insects.

Treatment.—Apply rags wetted with Goulard lotion (page 75). Look for the sting, and, if found, pull it out directly.

SNAKE BITES.—The bites of some snakes (as that of the cobra) are fatal to life, and others are highly dangerous. Lunar caustic, or a hot iron, should be immediately applied to the wounded part.

Brandy, or any other spirit, should be given in water frequently for several hours after the accident.

GUN-SHOT WOUNDS.—Bleeding from these wounds is the first evil to be remedied, and for this the same means are to be used as advised in the treatment under that heading (page 22).

(1) *Of the Head.*—If the ball enter the brain, immediate death almost always follows; but even when

the brain is injured and the skull broken, the patient will, under proper care, sometimes recover.

He must be kept perfectly quiet; the bleeding from the scalp need not be stopped directly. The loss of some blood will do good, and generally, when he becomes faint, the bleeding will cease.

The after-treatment will be low diet, purgatives, and cold to the head. The diet must be *low* for a fortnight at least, and on no account must any wine, beer, or spirits be given.

(2) *Of the Chest.*—The lungs may be wounded. In this case air and frothy blood often issue from the wound. The outward bleeding may be trifling, and the inward bleeding great.

Low diet only is to be given, consisting of toast and water, cold water, or a little beef-tea; and until the breathing is quite easy, he must live on slop food only. The state of the bowels must be watched, and wet lint should be placed over the wound.

(3) *Of the Belly.*—These are often fatal, as some vital part is generally wounded.

The patient must be placed on the wounded side, to allow the blood or other fluid to escape. Cold water, or toast and water *only*, should be taken, or he may suck ice or snow. An opium pill is to be given every four hours, until the patient becomes drowsy. The pills must then be left off until the drowsiness ceases, and again repeated. *No opening medicine must on any account be given.* Lint dipped in cold water should be applied to the wound.

WOUNDS OF JOINTS. These are serious injuries; and stiffness of the wounded parts, as well as severe pain and swelling, often follow. Wounds of the knee-joint are most common. The joint itself is known to be wounded when a clear yellowish fluid escapes, commonly called the joint oil.

Treatment.—A splint must be placed behind the injured joint, which should extend several inches above as well as below the joint, and be fitted with a pad. The wound must be closed at once by a piece of lint dipped in carbolic acid, which may be allowed to dry on and remain, and the limb must be kept quiet for three or four weeks.

PUTTING OUT OF JOINTS, OR DISLOCATIONS.

The joints most likely to be put out at sea are:

       (1) Shoulder.
       (2) Elbow.
       (3) Fingers.
       (4) Hip.
       (5) Ankle.

These accidents are easily repaired if taken in hand at once.

In all injuries of this kind, compare the sound limb with that which is hurt.

(1) SHOULDER.—There is flattening of the shoulder; a hollow is seen where there should be a rounded surface; the elbow sticks out from the side, and the

patient often holds it with the other hand to ease the pain; there is often great pain and numbness of fingers, and if you put your hand into the man's arm-pit, a round hard lump is felt.

Treatment.—Put the patient on his back, take off your boot, press your heel well into the arm-pit, seize the patient's hand, pull steadily, and the bone will slip into the socket with a loud snap. If the

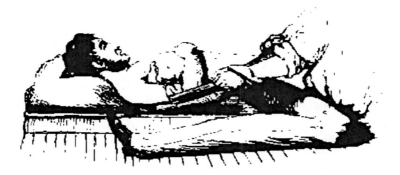

man be very muscular, a clove-hitch may be taken round the arm just above the elbow to aid a steady pull.

(2) ELBOW.—The arm is bent more or less at an angle, and cannot be straightened, and the bones are both felt and seen sticking out at the back part of the joint.

Treatment.—The patient having been seated, one man must take hold of the middle of the upper half of his arm, and another of his wrist. They must pull against each other, and a third should grasp the elbow with his two hands, his forefingers in front and his thumbs behind, with which he must press on the swelling downwards and forwards. After pulling some little time, bend the arm suddenly, and to the patient unexpectedly, and the bones will slip into their proper places.

Sometimes only one bone is out of place, which is thrown forwards, in which case the arm is slightly bent, but cannot be bent to a right angle, or completely straightened, and the palm of the hand is turned towards the body.

Treatment.—Pull in the same way as before indicated, and suddenly bend the elbow. The arm must be kept quiet in a sling for four or five days.

(3) FINGERS.—This injury is easily detected by the sticking out of the ends of the bones. It is repaired by fixing the displaced bone by a clove-hitch, and pulling steadily until the end slips into place.

This accident must be repaired at once, or great difficulty will afterwards be found in its management.

(4) THIGH-BONE.—The injured limb is from $1\frac{1}{2}$ to $2\frac{1}{2}$ inches shorter than the other, and the toe points inwards. The foot cannot be turned out, and any attempt to do so gives great pain; great pain is also given in separating the legs.

Treatment.—Pullies are often required to repair this accident. The patient must be laid on his back; the hip bones fixed by a stout piece of canvas passed between his legs and fastened to a staple in the deck, your heel pushed well up into the crutch, and a strong steady pull made by grasping the ankle with both hands. The repair may be assisted by placing a jack towel round the middle of the patient's thigh and round the neck of anyone who is helping you. Your assistant will then, by pulling gently, lift the head of the bone over the edge of the socket into its place. The bone will go in with a loud snap.

NOTE.—This accident is often difficult to discover, and you must therefore observe great caution in practising the above plan of treatment. If unsuccessful, do not persevere, but nurse the patient carefully until you arrive in port.

(5) ANKLE.—The lower end of the bone can be seen as a hard swelling and felt against the skin on the inner side of the ankle; there is a hollow on the outer side, and the sole of the foot is turned upwards and outwards.

Treatment.—Pull steadily until the foot is straight. A splint must then be placed on the inner side of the leg reaching above the knee, and below the ankle.

BROKEN BONES, OR FRACTURES.

These are of two classes, simple and compound.

A simple fracture is a broken bone with no wound.

A fracture is said to be compound when a wound leads from the skin to the broken bone.

BROKEN LOWER JAW.—Usually caused by a direct blow.

Symptoms.—On taking hold of the jaw with two hands, the broken ends can be felt grating against each other, and the regular line of the teeth is destroyed. The patient dribbles from the mouth, and speaks in a mumbling manner.

Treatment.—A piece of millboard, gutta percha, or *coarse* tarred felt, of this shape, is to be soaked in

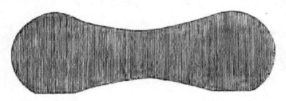

hot water, wrapped quickly in a piece of rag, the centre part placed under the chin, and the ends moulded, whilst soft, to the sides of the lower jaw. Each end of the splint should touch the lowest part of the ear, and, before soaking, it must be cut accordingly. It must be kept in its place by a four-tailed bandage thus—

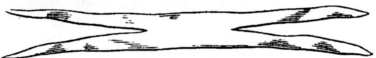

the two front tails being tied over the back and highest part of the head, in this way, and the hinder ones in front of them. The patient must be fed on slop diet for a fortnight after the accident.

BROKEN RIBS.—A sharp stabbing pain on taking breath, the patient often complaining that his ribs grate together; he will sometimes spit blood. On placing your hands over the painful spot, the ends of the broken bone may often be felt.

Treatment.—A flannel roller, seven inches wide, and seven yards long, must be tightly wound round the chest as high as the arms will permit.

GENERAL INDICATIONS OF BROKEN LIMBS.—Pain, inability to move the limb, and shortening, with grating of the broken ends.

BROKEN COLLAR-BONE.—The end of the bone is seen sticking up, the shoulder is flattened, and the patient cannot lift his arm to his head.

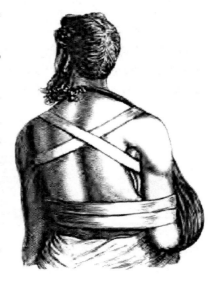

Treatment.—A bandage is to be applied round the shoulders thus, a large pad of cotton must be put in the arm pit, and the elbow pressed close to the side and supported in a sling.

BROKEN UPPER ARM (between shoulder-joint and elbow-joint).—The patient cannot move his arm, and there is deformity, with grating of the ends of the bone.

Treatment.—Bend the elbow, put on four splints, one inside, one outside, one in front, and one behind:

support the arm in a sling, and let the elbow be allowed to drop.

BROKEN LOWER ARM (between elbow-joint and wrist-joint)—All ordinary signs of a broken bone.

Treatment.—Bend the elbow, apply one splint on the inside of the arm reaching from the elbow to the tips of the fingers, and one on the outside reaching from the elbow to the back of the hand. The splints must be well padded.

BROKEN THIGH.—Shortening of the limb, turning out of the foot, with swelling of the foot, and grating of the broken ends of bone.

Treatment.—A well-padded long splint, extending from the arm-pit to the sole of the foot, is to be placed on the outside of the limb, the limb having

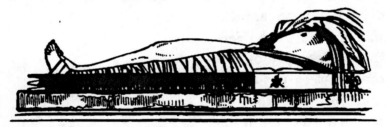

been first straightened by steady pulling; the splint must be fastened to the leg, thigh, and waist of the patient by leather straps, or by ordinary bandages. It must be kept on at least six weeks.

BROKEN LEG.—The same symptoms exist as in other ordinary fractures, viz. grating of bones, pain, and swelling.

Treatment.—A splint must be placed on each side

of the leg, reaching from above the knee to below the ankle, and fastened with bandages. The patient should generally be kept on his back, but the broken leg may, when carefully splintered and bandaged, be now and then laid on its side.

COMPOUND BROKEN BONES OR FRACTURES.

Treatment.—If the bone stick out of the wound, it must be put back, which can generally be done by steady pulling; but if the bone be jammed, it will be necessary to enlarge the wound with a lancet, and a piece of lint dipped in the blood should then be applied over the wound, and allowed to dry on. Two side splints, one on either side of the limb, must be applied, and the limb kept cool by a wet rag.

In the treatment of all fractures, rest is of very great importance, and the limb, when once set, should be disturbed as little as possible, unless the splints have shifted. All patients with broken bones should, if possible, be put into a sling cot, and *all splints should be kept on for five weeks.*

BRUISES.

BRUISES are too well known to need description, and need no treatment unless very severe.

Treatment.—Rags wetted with Goulard lotion (page 75) should be applied, or hot fomentations used if cold is disagreeable.

BLEEDING.

It is very important to act promptly when a patient is bleeding from a wound, and a different plan must be followed according as the blood flows from an artery or vein. The blood from an artery is of a bright red colour, and that from a vein bluish and dark. Bleeding may always be controlled for a time by pressure. A firm pad of lint should be placed over the bleeding spot, pressed and kept in its place by plaster. If this be insufficient, pressure should be applied by the fingers, and the part should be kept cold by ice, snow, or a stream of cold water. If the bleeding still continue, and be bright red and jerking, and the seat of injury be the arm or leg, pressure must be made over the principal artery of the part. This can generally be felt beating on *the inside* of the limb; and a bandage must be

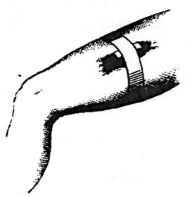

fixed thus, placed on the spot where the artery feels to be nearest the surface, and tightened until the bleeding ceases. If a vein burst, or be cut, and if the injury be in the leg, the patient must at once lie down.

Bleeding from a vein is always easily stopped by the pressure of a pad. No pressure *above* the wound should be made in this case, as it will greatly increase the bleeding.

Directions for making a Pad.—It should be about an inch thick, and made of several layers of lint or rag, of various sizes. The smallest piece is to be placed over the wound, from which the blood has been carefully wiped, and the rest in order of size. A piece of cork wrapped in lint is to be put on the top of the pad, and the whole arrangement fastened by a piece of plaster or a bandage.

If the wound be in the arm or leg, the limb must be raised to assist the return of blood.

GATHERING, OR ABSCESS.

This is generally caused by a blow or strain, and is a hot and painful swelling, at first hard, but eventually bursting, and discharging matter.

Treatment.—A linseed-meal poultice, which must be changed twice a day.

When the swelling softens, and the skin over it is red and very thin, time will be gained and suffering saved by opening it with a lancet. Continue the poultice after the abscess is opened. When the skin is very thick, as in the palm of the hand and over the fingers, it will separate, and should be cut away with a pair of scissors.

BURNS AND SCALDS.

Treatment.—In slight cases, a thick layer of flour

should be dusted over the part, so as to form a crust, beneath which, if not very deep, the burn will heal.

In severe cases, pieces of rag should be dipped in oil, placed on the burn, and covered with cotton wool; the dressings must be changed as seldom as possible, but sufficiently often to ensure cleanliness, and must then be gently washed off with carbolic acid lotion (page 76). The patient's strength must be supported by good food, and a daily allowance of grog, and the pain relieved by a draught at night containing 40 drops of laudanum.

Burns of the face are best treated by painting on olive oil with a soft brush, or with the feather of a pen.

If large blisters form, they should be pricked with a needle and covered with flour and cotton wool. The wrinkled skin must not be cut off.

INJURIES TO THE HEAD.

Common among sailors, and often of a serious nature.

Wounds of the scalp, even if small, may be followed by very awkward consequences; and, indeed, no injury of the head, however slight, should be neglected.

These wounds may be clean-cut or jagged, and in any case bleed freely.

Treatment.—Shave the part, clean the wound, and, if large, bring the edges together by one or two stitches. A pad of lint kept in its place by plaster is a sufficient covering, and the bleeding is always easily stopped by pressure with fingers or bandage.

In all injuries of this kind the patient must be kept on *low* diet, and his bowels must be freely opened. If he complains of headache, or is drowsy, cut his hair short, and put rags wetted with cold water to his scalp. *No wine, beer, or spirits must on any account be given.*

CONCUSSION OR CONFUSION OF THE BRAIN.—This is a consequence of severe blows on the head or of falls from aloft, and the scalp is sometimes wounded.

The patient in a slight case is faint, feels sick, and sometimes vomits.

If the injury be severe, he loses his senses; his body is cold; he lies as if in a deep sleep, but can be roused by shouting some familiar question in his ear, when he will answer, and immediately go off to sleep again. This drowsiness may last from one to forty-eight hours.

Treatment.—Keep him quiet; give nothing, or you may choke him; wrap him in a warm blanket, and apply warmth to his feet.

BROKEN SKULL AND PRESSURE ON THE BRAIN.— Generally a fatal accident.

The patient is insensible, breathes as if smoking a pipe, and sometimes bleeds at the ears and nose.

Treatment.—Apply cold to the head and warmth to the feet. Nothing else can be done.

FROST BITE.

This accident occurs most commonly to coloured seamen, and affects the fingers and toes. Urge your men, when the ship is in cold latitudes, to come to you as soon as their extremities become red or at all shrunken.

Treatment.—Rub the parts affected with snow or ice, and afterwards apply rags wetted with cold water. Do not bring the patient into a warm cabin, or near a fire, or the limb may be destroyed.

HANGING.

Cut the patient down, make everything clear about the neck, and dash cold water on the face and chest. If necessary, employ directions given in the article on drowning (see below).

DROWNING.

Take off all clothes at once, wipe the body dry, rub it well with hot cloths, and put hot bottles into the armpits, between the calves of the legs, and to the feet; wipe the mouth and nostrils, excite breathing by tickling the throat with a feather, keep up the rubbing for several hours with relays of hands, and you may save life when all means used for its restoration appear hopeless.

In addition to these directions, the following are copied from those of the National Lifeboat Institution, and are most valuable *if properly practised*:—

To Restore Breathing.

To Clear the Throat.—Place the patient on the floor or ground with the face downwards, and one of the arms under the forehead, in which position all fluids will more readily escape by the mouth, and the tongue itself will fall forward, leaving the entrance into the windpipe free. Assist this operation by wiping and cleansing the mouth.

If satisfactory breathing commences, use the treatment described below to promote warmth. If there be only slight breathing—or no breathing—or if the breathing fail, then—

To Excite Breathing—Turn the patient well and instantly on the side, supporting the head, and excite the nostrils with snuff, hartshorn, and smelling salts, or tickle the throat with a feather, &c., if they are at hand. Rub the chest and face warm, and dash cold water, or cold and hot water alternately, on them If there be no success, lose not a moment, but instantly—

To Imitate Breathing—Replace the patient on the face, raising and supporting the chest well on a folded coat or other article of dress.

Turn the body very gently on the side, and a little beyond, and then briskly on the face, back again, repeating these measures cautiously, efficiently, and perseveringly, about fifteen times in the minute, or once every four or five seconds, occasionally varying the side.

By placing the patient on the chest, the weight of the body forces the air out; when turned on the side, this pressure is removed, and air enters the chest.

On each occasion that the body is replaced on the face, make uniform but efficient pressure with brisk movement, on the back between and below the shoulder-blades or bones on each side, removing the pressure immediately before turning the body on the side.

During the whole of the operations let one person attend solely to the movements of the head and of the arm placed under it.

The first measure increases the expiration—the second commences inspiration.

Should these efforts not prove successful in the course of from two to five minutes, proceed to imitate breathing by Dr. SILVESTER'S method, as follows:—

Place the patient on the back on a flat surface, inclined a little upwards from the feet; raise and support the head and shoulders on a small firm cushion or folded article of dress placed under the shoulder-blades.

Draw forward the patient's tongue, and keep it projecting beyond the lips: an elastic band over the tongue and under the chin will answer this purpose, or a piece of string or tape may be tied round them, or by raising the lower jaw, the teeth may be made to retain the tongue in that position. Remove all tight clothing from about the neck and chest, especially the braces.

To imitate the Movements of Breathing.—Standing at the patient's head, grasp the arms just above the elbows, and draw the arms gently and steadily upwards above the head, and *keep them stretched* upwards for two seconds. (*By this means air is drawn into the lungs.*) Then turn down the patient's arms, and press them gently and firmly for two seconds against the sides of the chest. (*By this means air is pressed out of the lungs.*)

Repeat these measures alternately, deliberately, and perseveringly, about fifteen times in a minute, until a spontaneous effort to respire is perceived, immediately upon which cease to imitate the movements of breathing, and proceed to *Induce Circulation and Warmth.*

The above treatment should be persevered in for some hours, as it is an erroneous opinion that persons are irrecoverable because life does not soon make its appearance, persons having been restored after persevering for many hours.

Cautions.—Prevent unnecessary crowding of persons round the body, especially if in an apartment.

Avoid rough usage, and do not allow the body to remain on the back unless the tongue is secured.

Under no circumstances hold the body up by the feet.

When consciousness returns, give the patient light fluid food, with a little wine, and let him rest completely for at least twenty-four hours, or he may have a severe fever, and will then be confined to his berth for some weeks.

CHOKING, OR SUFFOCATION.

Commonly caused by breathing foul air of any kind.

Bring the patient at once into fresh air, and treat him by the directions given under the heads of hanging and drowning (see page 26).

FAINTING.

This may occur from loss of blood, from fatigue, or from excessive weakness produced by any exhausting disease.

Treatment.—The patient must be laid down, *with his head as low as the rest of the body.* Give him plenty of air, and sprinkle cold water smartly over his face and chest.

POISONS.

TAKE CARE to find out what the patient has swallowed, as, in cases of poisoning, an improper remedy is far worse than none at all.

ACIDS,
AS, SPIRIT OF SALTS, AQUA-FORTIS, &c.

Give bi-carbonate of soda in water, chalk or whiting in water, or if neither of these be at hand, *soap suds.*

Give an ounce of castor oil afterwards to open the bowels, and repeat it the next day.

POTASHES, HARTSHORN, AND AMMONIA.

Give vinegar and water. After-treatment as for acids.

LEAD.

Give Epsom salts in large quantities, which should be continued in doses sufficiently strong to keep the bowels freely open three days after all active symptoms of poisoning have passed away.

OPIUM, OR LAUDANUM.

There is no antidote for this poison.

If the patient will swallow anything, give him 30 grains of sulphate of zinc in a large glass of water, make him drink large quantities of water, and tickle his throat with a feather, to make him vomit.

He must be kept awake at any cost, by splashing with cold water, and must be walked about until all symptoms of profound drowsiness have vanished. Give him strong coffee often, but in small quantities, keep him warm, and when he is thoroughly awakened, let him have a short sleep of about thirty or forty minutes, then get the bowels open with a full dose (1½ oz.) of castor oil, and keep up warmth of body, if necessary, by rubbing and hot bottles.

ARSENIC.

If no vomiting has occurred, give the man 30 grains of sulphate of zinc in a large glass of water, or, if this be not close at hand, a large draught of very greasy water, or of warm sea water, and repeat it until he vomits. If this does not succeed quickly, the patient will probably die.

FISH-POISONING.

This accident occurs now and then on board ship. Give your patient 30 grains of sulphate of zinc in a large glass of water to make him vomit, and let him have afterwards small and oft-repeated doses of brandy.

EXCESSIVE DRUNKENNESS.

Give the man 30 grains of sulphate of zinc in a glass of beer, or any other liquid, to make him vomit. Get everything clear about his neck and waist, rest his head, well raised, on a wet swab, and put him in the open air, properly protected from cold.

TAKE NOTICE.

In all cases of poisoning, your remedies should be found at once, and given speedily, with little or no special care as to the quantity administered, and you need not be surprised if the patient is unfit for work for several days after the occurrence.

MEDICAL DISEASES.

The term 'slop diet' is used to signify any kind of food in a fluid state, as beef tea, soups, milk, arrowroot, &c.

FEVER.

BY fever is not meant ague, but a continued state of hot skin, furred or dry tongue, with very loose or very confined bowels.

There are many varieties of fever, but these three may be distinguished without much difficulty.

(1) Heat of skin, loss of appetite, tongue sometimes dry, sometimes furred and moist, bowels generally confined.

This lasts from one to six days.

Give your patient an ounce of castor oil if he requires it, the fever mixture (page 74) three times a day, and slop diet, and when the fever has left him, two grains of quinine three times a day for a week, with good diet.

(2) A moist furred tongue, hot skin, loose bowels, and tight belly, sounding, when gently tapped, like a drum.

This will continue for three weeks.

Put a large turpentine fomentation (page 76) over his stomach, keep it there for thirty minutes, and repeat it every morning for three days successively if the looseness continue. Give him a dose of paregoric three times a day, and six grains of Dover's powder every night. Keep him up with all the good broth and slop diet that you can command, and if his tongue become hard and dry, give him wine, or brandy and water at the rate of from 4 oz. to 12 oz. of brandy every twenty-four hours. If the looseness is very bad (say from twelve to twenty stools in twenty-four hours), give him the diarrhœa mixture (page 74) every four hours, but knock it off directly the diarrhœa moderates, as a certain amount of looseness assists to get rid of this disease.

(3) A leathery dry tongue, hot skin, and confined bowels, with occasional and sometimes violent wanderings.

This will continue for two weeks.

Shave the head, and apply cold; get the bowels open as quickly, and keep them open as regularly, as possible; give very good nourishing slop food, very often, but in small quantities; and begin at once with 6 oz. of brandy every twenty-four hours, increasing it to 12 oz. if the pulse is very feeble; but when the tongue becomes soft and less dry, you may knock off half the brandy.

In all these varieties of fever—

(1) See that the patient makes water, and if he does not do so, use the catheter very gently every twelve hours (directions for use of catheter at page 60).

(2) Keep him very clean and dry, or he will get bedsores.

(3) Give no medicines except those indicated above.

These forms of fever (with scarlet fever elsewhere described) require more attention than any other disease, and the life of your patient will generally depend on the care and watchfulness of the nurse, doctoring being of very little service.

AGUE, OR INTERMITTENT FEVER.

This disease, in one form or other, occurs chiefly in China, the West Indies, and on the west coast of Africa. A violent chill, followed by great heat, the whole attack lasting from two to eight hours, are sufficiently distinct symptoms, and two things are to be done before you can commence any satisfactory treatment—1st. See that the bowels are well opened with a dose of black draught; 2ndly. Find out as exactly as is possible the hour at which the chill fit usually begins.

This will, with some care, be almost always ascertained. Having succeeded in fixing the time, give your patient 10 grains of quinine in a little water two hours before the expected attack. Repeat this twice, and, if unsuccessful in stopping the fit, or lessening its severity, increase the dose to 15 grains. Having stopped the chill fit completely, keep up this large dose three times afterwards, two hours before the expected attack, and give the man, besides these large doses, 3 grains of quinine three times a day, making him take this last prescription at least a week after all signs of the disease have passed away.

SCARLET FEVER, SMALL-POX, MEASLES, AND ERYSIPELAS.

These diseases, happily, seldom occur on board ship; but it is necessary that they should be mentioned in this book, and they are grouped together because their early symptoms are the same, and, with the exception of erysipelas, you must treat them all in precisely the same manner.

SCARLET FEVER is known by a sore red throat, a strawberry-red tongue, and a scarlet rash on the body.

It lasts from eight to ten days.

SMALL-POX is too well known to need any description here, though it is sometimes confounded with spots which are caused by venereal disease.

It lasts from sixteen to twenty days.

MEASLES commence with sneezing, snuffling, and a running at the eyes, soon after which clusters of large spots appear, first on the face, and afterwards on the lower parts of the body. They feel 'shotty,' and raised to the touch.

The disease lasts from five to ten days.

ERYSIPELAS is known by an intensely red and shiny condition of the skin, which begins by a single spot, extends very rapidly, produces much swelling, and (except in the case of wounds) nearly always appears on the face, scalp, or legs.

It lasts from three to ten days.

All these maladies commence with wandering pains in the back, and a varying amount of general fever.

Keep the bowels gently open; give the fever mixture (page 74) three times a day; and if the man's tongue become dry, or if he begin to wander, put him on an allowance of from 6 oz. to 12 oz. of rum or brandy every twenty-four hours, knocking it off as these latter symptoms disappear.

In cases of erysipelas, wrap up the part affected in cotton-wool, or powder it well from the cook's dredging-box with flour, or if you have neither wool nor flour, cover it up lightly with tow, to keep the air out as much as possible.

All these patients want good slop diet, and it is your duty to caution them, when recovering, against getting wet, or remaining in wet clothes one minute longer than is necessary. Dropsy and other disorders may come on, and carelessness as to this simple point has lost the lives of many men on shore as well as afloat.

It is proper to remind you that these four diseases are all very decidedly catching; that, though it may be impossible on board ship to house sick men apart from the rest, you will consult the health and safety of all by putting such patients by themselves as far as is practicable.

Wash and swab out their quarters with carbolic acid water every morning, keep them very clean, and, when they are well, throw overboard their beds and bedding, if you can possibly afford to do so.

YELLOW FEVER.

This disease exists only in countries where the temperature reaches at least 75 degrees Fahr^t. It occurs chiefly in the West Indies, in those parts of the Americas bordering on the Gulf of Mexico, on the west coast of Africa, and sometimes in Spain.

Its chief symptoms are well known to all who have frequented the coasts above mentioned, and are yellowness of the skin, intense fever, and the vomiting of a dark-brown fluid.

This disease lasts from ten to thirty days, and if the patient survives to the fifth day, the case is generally hopeful. Get the bowels open as speedily and as thoroughly as possible with full doses of castor oil. Shave the head, and apply cold to it constantly. Sponge the body with cold water if the heat of skin continue; but if the patient becomes cold, as is sometimes the case, put him into a warm bath at a temperature of 90 degrees.

Give the fever mixture (page 74) three times a day, and if he is excessively restless, an opium pill at night, with very good slop diet at frequent intervals both night and day.

Keep him very clean; see that he makes water regularly, and use the catheter if necessary (page 60).

When the heat of skin and other serious symptoms have passed away, let his rations be as good and liberal as possible, with a daily allowance of wine or beer, and give him 3 grains of quinine three times a.day for a fortnight.

COUGH, BRONCHITIS, INFLAMMATION OF THE LUNGS, AND CONSUMPTION.

(1) A severe cough, with a variable quantity of frothy, white, and sometimes mattery expectoration, will generally indicate bronchitis, which lasts from five to ten days.

(2) A cough, with a small quantity of rusty or bloody expectoration, much heat of skin, and difficulty of breathing, will generally indicate inflammation of the lungs, which lasts from four to nine days.

(3) A lasting cough, with much mattery and often bad-smelling expectoration, often accompanied by occasional attacks of blood-spitting, as well as by loss of flesh and debility, will indicate consumption.

(1) For the first of these, keep the man warm, and his bowels gently open; put warm fomentations to his chest, and, if he gets no sleep at all, give him a

cough pill now and then at night, and the fever mixture (page 74) three times a day.

(2) For the second, pursue the same course, and give in addition from 4 oz. to 12 oz. of brandy every twenty-four hours until the spitting ceases to be rusty, and the skin to be hot. Put a linseed-meal poultice to that part of the chest where the pain is most felt, and change it every six hours. Tell off the very best man that you have to nurse him; give him very good slop diet, and you will save life in many cases.

(3) For the third, pursue the same plan as for the first; give the cough pill, if it relieves pain, every other night, and, if the violent symptoms subside, let him have as much fresh air and good diet as possible.

No medicines that you can give are of any service beyond those above indicated.

QUINSY.

A swelling of one or both tonsils (which are small round lumps at the back of the throat) is a sufficient explanation of this disease, which is often very alarming and very distressing to the patient, but rarely fatal.

It lasts from five to ten days.

Get the bowels open, and make him gargle continually with warm water. After much pain, and apparent danger of suffocation, the swelling will burst, and the man will speedily get well.

HEART DISEASES.

Heart diseases are mostly difficult to discover. The general symptoms are shortness of breath, with or without cough, pain about the left nipple, with palpitation, and a swelling of the legs, purse, and sometimes of the body, commonly called dropsy. (Dropsy, however, often exists in diseases of the liver and of the kidneys.)

If there is much pain, put a hot fomentation on the chest, and if the dropsy increases, get the bowels freely open with a dose of cream of tartar, in a little water, repeating this every third day for about fourteen days, if it does not appear to weaken the patient. *Opium must not be given* in these cases to procure sleep, and very little can be done, as nearly all varieties of heart disease are incurable.

If any spitting of blood occur, nothing warm must be taken.

JAUNDICE, AND LIVER DISEASES.

Jaundice, like cough and diarrhœa, is only a sign of disease, and as a cough shows that something is wrong with the lungs, and diarrhœa points to cholera, fever, or dysentery, so jaundice shows that the liver is out of order.

Yellowness of the skin and of the eyes is a sufficient indication of jaundice, which may accompany any form of liver disease.

These forms of disease are so various and intricate that a detailed description of them would be confusing and useless. You must therefore treat symptoms.

In all cases give one of the strong or mild purging pills, and half a blue pill, every night for four nights running. If there be much pain over the liver, put on a turpentine fomentation (page 76) once or twice only, and, if the pain be intensely severe and come on suddenly, give an opium pill, but do not repeat it unless absolutely necessary.

Most disorders of the liver are known by a pain in the right shoulder, a dull aching on the right side, sluggishness of the bowels, and excessive general weakness.

Some forms of liver disease are caused by drinking, some by dysentery, and some by the passage of a gallstone; but you cannot do more than that above indicated, and you will find, after reaching temperate latitudes, that the patient will generally improve.

CONSTIPATION.

An obstinate confinement of the bowels is often aggravated rather than relieved by the use of purgatives. Give two compound rhubarb pills every other night for a week; if this does not succeed, an injection up the vent of soap and water, or weigh out 80 grains of soap, knead it well, and tell the patient to pass it cautiously into the vent. *Ask every man who complains of constipation if he has a rupture*, and, if this be the case, treat him immediately as directed in this book (see page 58). Do not persevere with purgatives if the above directions fail; give any sort of fruits (fresh or preserved) if you have them on board, tell the patient to take a cold bath every morning, and leave the rest to nature.

INDIGESTION.

This is a very common complaint among sailors, who will come aft complaining of wind on the stomach and pain about the belly after meals. Give the stomachic mixture (page 75) twice a day, and a mild purging pill, if necessary, for three nights in succession.

DIARRHŒA.

Sailors are often attacked with simple looseness of the bowels, but when an illness begins in this way, look out for fever (as described in page 34), dysentery (page 46), or cholera (page 45). If you cannot satisfy yourself that the looseness is a symptom of any of these diseases, and you believe that the diarrhœa arises from something injurious that has been swallowed by the patient, let it go on for some hours, and put your patient on slop diet. But if it continue beyond four or five hours, give him a dose of the diarrhœa powder (page 72) after every loose motion, and he will soon get perfectly well.

But in all places where cholera is known to exist, and no doctor is near, urge your men strongly to come aft directly any diarrhœa commences, and *give them the diarrhœa powder after every loose motion until the looseness has ceased.*

Strict attention to these directions may save many lives.

CHOLERA.

This disease generally commences with simple diarrhœa, which may go on from two to eight days. If neglected, agonising cramps, stools resembling rice-water, vomiting, and a general blueness of the body follow.

This stage lasts from two to forty-eight hours.

If the patient survive it, he will either improve very rapidly, or will have an attack of fever, with hot skin, white furred tongue, and great general weakness.

This stage lasts from two to seven days.

It cannot be too forcibly impressed upon your mind that no good can be done unless you treat a case in the first stage, and so I repeat a warning before mentioned—that you should urge upon all your men to come aft as soon as any looseness of the bowels begins. Give them the diarrhœa mixture (page 74) after every loose motion, doubling the dose if necessary, and, above all, let them have as much rest as you can.

Throw overboard all stools passed, and, if possible, all soiled clothes, and wash out the quarters where the patient is berthed frequently with carbolic acid water.

Medicines are useless in the second stage (cramps, &c.); so keep the patient as warm as possible, and give him as much cold water as he wishes to drink.

Give no medicine in the third stage (fever), but keep up the patient's strength with as good a diet as you have.

DYSENTERY.

This disease is almost entirely confined to the crews of ships trading to China and the East Indies; sometimes, but much more rarely, it occurs in those coming from the West Indies, west coast of Africa, South America, and some of the Mediterranean ports, particularly Alexandria and Odessa.

The symptoms are well known to most captains:—

Looseness of the bowels, with much straining, stools more or less bloody, resulting in great general weakness.

In nine-tenths of the cases that occur in East India and China ships, the sailors will tell you that they had dysentery in the country before sailing, and this probably for some weeks. If such a history be made out satisfactorily, you must let your patient have as much rest as possible, give him slop diet, continue his limejuice, let him have 10 grains of Dover's powder three times a day, 10 drops of laudanum in an ounce of castor oil every third day, and plenty of warmth to the body. Leave off the limejuice at the end of a week for a few days only, if it appears to aggravate the disease, *but under no other circumstances.* This is the only useful treatment for such cases in the tropical seas; you will find that, when temperate latitudes are reached, your patient will

almost invariably improve; and you may then give
him 2 grains of quinine three times a day for several
weeks. Arrowroot, sago, flour, rice, or any other
light extras that you may have, are always well
expended on such cases. If, however, you are
perfectly satisfied that the disease has commenced
for the first time in a man *after* the ship has
put to sea, pursue the same directions as to diet,
knock off all his limejuice, and instead of Dover's
powder, give 5 grains of ipecacuanha powder three
times a day, gradually increasing the dose to 10 or
15 grains if no vomiting occur. If your patient
does not improve under this treatment, give him his
limejuice again, and pursue the same plan as that
first recommended. It must be recollected, however, that in India and China very few cases of
dysentery *commence* after leaving port, the vast
majority being cases where the disease has begun
during the sailor's stay in the country.

No other patients that may come under your care
will so well repay all possible indulgence that you can
give them in the matter of rest when ill, and easy
deck work when improving.

COLIC.

This disease frequently occurs among seamen and
others from no very obvious cause, and also after
drinking water that has passed through leaden pipes,
or has been kept in leaden vessels; or more often

breaks out among a ship's crew after working at any occupation in which white or red lead is used. It begins with severe twisting pains about the belly, which is not tender on pressure. The pains commence suddenly, and come on again at irregular intervals, with great confinement of the bowels. Look for a narrow blue line along the edge of the gums, which, if found, is at once a proof that lead is the cause of the disease. It is probable that several of the crew will be affected at the same time. If this be the case, and you are using white or any other kind of lead in painting or repairing the ship, leave off the work as soon as is practicable. Give your patients a good dose of castor oil with 10 drops of laudanum, put them on slop diet, and make them wash themselves and their clothes thoroughly. When the bowels have acted well, give them a dose of salts and nitrate of potash, with essence of ginger, twice a day, and, if the pain continue, put on their stomachs a large hot fomentation, repeating this until the pain abates. This treatment, *with entire absence from all work in which lead is used,* must be continued until the bowels are regular and the patient free from pain, or palsy of the hands may follow, and the men will then be entirely useless to you for the rest of the voyage.

KIDNEY DISEASES.

These maladies are difficult to detect, and their symptoms by no means easy to describe.

Pain in the loins, great general depression, and (as with heart disease) great general dropsy, are the chief and only marked signs.

If the patient be tolerably strong, keep the bowels very freely open for fourteen days by giving a dose of cream of tartar, in a little water, every other morning. Should the swelling not be reduced, or the pain relieved, by this treatment, you can do nothing more to aid strength except by feeding the man tolerably well.

Heart and kidney affections are the most hopeless kinds of internal diseases, and in the vast majority of cases your patients will be fit for no more active work than sailmaking, cleaning brass-work, quartermaster's duty, or giving a hand to the cook.

FITS.

In all kinds of fits commonly so called, observe strictly the following rules :—

(1) Give the man plenty of air, and loosen all clothes about the neck and body.

(2) Do not attempt to make him swallow anything at all, until you are convinced that he is sensible.

(3) Do not use more violence than is absolutely necessary in restraining struggling movements.

No other rules are required for your guidance, whatever the fit may be.

When it is over, get the bowels open, keep the man quiet, and put him on slop diet for twenty-four hours.

SUNSTROKE.

Send your patient at once into the coolest place that you can find, get his head shaved, pour cold water over the head, and dash it smartly and frequently over the head, neck, and chest, and give an ounce of castor oil immediately, repeating the dose, until the bowels are freely and thoroughly relieved, four or five times; keep him quiet and on slop diet for at least two days after, and see that his head is always covered when on deck.

PALSY.

Loss of power in arms, legs, bladder, and, in fact, any part of the body, occurring as a consequence of many other diseases.

You can do nothing by active medicine, but it is your duty to see that he is kept as clean as possible, so as to avoid bedsores; that his bowels are regularly relieved, and that his food is good. No stimulants are necessary. Ask him if he passes urine regularly. If none passes for twenty hours, and a warm bath fails to relieve him, you must use the catheter (page 60), taking care to pull out the wire before introducing the instrument into the yard.

DELIRIUM TREMENS.

This disease will not very often come under your notice, but its mention is necessary, as you may be called upon to treat a patient soon after getting out of port.

Inability to sleep, want of appetite, and restlessness, amounting to temporary, and even violent, madness, are, with an easily discovered history of drinking, sufficient indications of this disease. The first necessary step is to get a free action of the bowels. ·Give a large black draught, and repeat it in six hours, if necessary. Keep a constant watch over the patient if he is at all restless, and do not use more actual restraint than is necessary for the man's safety and that of others around him. If you are very short of hands, and the man is exceedingly and continuously violent, give him a grain of opium, and repeat it, if no effect be produced, in two hours; but opium is a dangerous medicine in this disease, and should not be given unless you believe that the man will die from exhaustion, or unless you cannot spare hands to watch him without endangering the safety of the ship.

No after-treatment is required.

SCURVY.

Swollen and spongy gums, dark spots and blue blotches, like bruises, about the legs, and a brawny hardness about the calves of the legs and under parts of the thighs, are the outward and visible signs of this disease.

Double the man's daily allowance of limejuice, and give him any kind of vegetables, preserved or otherwise, that you have on board, with a liberal allowance of pickles, beer or wine.

If the provisions of The Merchant Shipping Act of 1867 be faithfully carried out by the government, as well as by your owners and yourselves, scurvy will soon be an unknown disease in the merchant navy of this country; and if the article in this book headed 'Prevention of Disease' be strictly followed, no serious outbreak of scurvy need be feared by the captain of any ship.

RHEUMATISM.

Rheumatism may be caused by exposure to cold and wet, or may be the result of pox or clap. No description of this disease is needed, but it is sometimes so severe as to render the patient quite helpless, and is then called acute rheumatism, which lasts from fourteen to twenty days.

If a man be attacked with this last form of the disease, keep him very warm, and wrap up the joints affected in flannel. Get the bowels open, and, if there is very much pain, give him 10 grains of Dover's powder every night, and the saline mixture (page 74) three times a day. You must move him very gently indeed, and meddle with his limbs in doing so as little as possible, for the pain of a rheumatic joint, when roughly handled, is horrible to bear.

For all other kinds of rheumatism, use the saline mixture (page 74) three times a day, and make your patient clothe warmly; you will often cut short his illness by several weeks, and make him quickly useful, if you let him turn in for one or two whole nights, and give him, when in his berth, 10 grains of Dover's powder, with a stiff glass of hot grog.

Rheumatism is, however, often very obstinate, and more sailors are permanently disabled year by year from this, than from any other, disease.

The provisions of the Merchant Shipping Act, 1867, require all sleeping places to be dry and well ventilated, and will, with dry clothes and dry bedding, *prevent* more rheumatism than any captain, mate, or doctor can possibly cure.

ITCH.

This disease is caused by dirty habits as to clothes and person.

The spots, which are sometimes like small bladders of water, usually commence between the fingers, but soon spread indifferently over any part of the body, particularly the arms, legs, and buttocks.

After the patient has washed well with soft soap and warm water, make him smear all parts of the skin affected with the sulphur ointment (page 76), and keep him in a greasy state until all sense of itching or a desire to scratch has passed away.

The man should, as far as is practicable, lie apart from the rest of the crew. Burn all his bedding and greasy clothes when he is well, if you can afford to do so, as you may thereby save a round of the disease among your hands.

SURGICAL DISEASES.

VENEREAL DISEASES.

THESE include :—

    (1) External Clap.
    (2) Gonorrhea or Clap.
    (3) Chafes.
    (4) Chancre.
    (5) Bubo.

There are also other complaints which may follow at a later period. Swelled testicle often follows clap; spots and ulcers on the skin, and sore throat, often follow chancre.

(1) EXTERNAL CLAP.—This is a common disease with men who have long foreskins. It arises from uncleanliness. Dirt collects under the foreskin, and irritates the glans penis or nut.

A thick discharge comes from under the foreskin, which is swollen and drawn back with difficulty. The nut is red and swollen, but there is no ulcer.

The foreskin must be well pulled back, and it, as well as the nut, washed with warm water. Both must then be swabbed with the caustic lotion (page 75). A piece of lint should then be placed between the nut and foreskin, and the foreskin drawn forward into its proper place.

Attention to cleanliness for a few days, with repetition, if necessary, of the swabbing, will effect a speedy cure.

(2) CLAP.—This disease generally appears from two days to a week after connection with a foul woman.

Symptoms.—There is itching at the end of the passage through which the urine flows; the nut also swells, and its skin has a red shiny look; there is a feeling of heat and smarting when passing water, which soon amounts to scalding, and sometimes causes great pain. The stream of urine is twisted and broken, and in bad cases may stop altogether. Then follows a greenish-yellow discharge, at first thin, but afterwards thick and mattery. There is also a sense of itching along the under surface of the yard in the direction of the vent, and the patient is often troubled by painful erections at night. If the foreskin be long, and the discharge from the passage allowed to collect underneath, the foreskin swells, cannot be drawn back, and external clap, as well as ordinary clap, appears.

Treatment.—Give a purging pill, followed by a dose of salts or a black draught, and repeat this dose if necessary. The injection of the sulphate of zinc (page 76) should be used twice a day; and if, after the expiration of a week or ten days, no improvement takes place, the copaiba mixture (page 75) should be given three times a day.

How to use the Injection.—A squirt is to be filled with the injection, the end of this squirt put into the passage as far as it will go, and the injection then slowly and steadily squirted into the yard. When the squirt is taken away, the passage should be closed by the finger and thumb for a few seconds to keep in the injection.

LESSER DISORDERS WHICH MAY FOLLOW CLAP.

ERECTIONS.—The yard should be soaked in water as hot as can be borne for twenty minutes before turning in. If the erections occur in spite of these precautions, the pain is relieved by sitting on cold metal, or by sluicing the yard well with cold water, and by giving a double dose of the soothing mixture (page 74) every night.

RETENTION OF URINE. See page 60.

SWELLED TESTICLE.—The patient has pain and a sense of weight in the testicle, and pain up the cord. The testicle soon increases to two or three times its natural size, and becomes very tender. There is also a feeling of sickness, and of pain in the loins, furred tongue, confined bowels, and general fever.

Treatment.—A good purge, and the soothing mixture (page 74) three times a day. The testicle must be well kept up by a bandage or handkerchief, and the patient must, if possible, knock off work, as rest is very important. Put hot fomentations to the testicle, or a hot linseed-meal poultice, with which a teaspoonful of laudanum should be mixed. Warmth is generally preferred to cold; but if cold appear to give more relief, apply a lotion made with Goulard extract and laudanum (page 75). Barley-water, linseed-tea, or toast and water should be given. A bandage to keep up the testicle should be worn for two or three months.

(3) CHAFES.—These are sores on the surface, generally caused by dirt. They mostly appear in the groove between the foreskin and the nut, are of small size, and easily cured.

Treatment.—Wash well with warm water, use the caustic lotion (page 75), and apply dry lint.

(4) CHANCRE.—This begins as a small pimple, which itches a good deal; a watery head then forms, which bursts and leaves a sore. Chancres may be hard or soft. The hard chancre has a gristly edge, and is best treated, and must be kept constantly wetted, with black wash. The soft chancre only requires to be kept clean, and touched occasionally with caustic.

Mercury should not be given at all by an unprofessional person. All venereal sores will heal without mercury, if the directions given above are strictly followed.

Chancres are often followed by sore throat, spots on the skin, pains in, and swellings on, the bones, and ulcers.

Give all such cases 5 grains of iodide of potassium in a little water three times a day for several weeks;

let them wash out their throats with the gargle (page 75), and dress the ulcers carefully with simple ointment. Give them also a double allowance of limejuice daily, *to prevent the great tendency to scurvy that exists in all these patients.*

(5) BUBO.—A swelling in the groin, which becomes red, softens, and, if left to itself, bursts, and discharges matter by a small hole.

Treatment.—Hot linseed-meal poultices and rest; when the skin becomes very thin, the bubo may be opened. This should be done by lancing the swelling *across, not lengthways*; the poultice should be continued for two or three days afterwards, and should be followed by lint and water dressing or carbolic acid lotion. The bowels must be kept open with occasional purgatives, and after the bubo has burst, or been opened, you should help on the man's strength by good food and a small quantity of wine, beer, or grog.

RUPTURE.

This is a common affection among sailors, on account of the violent exertions undergone in hauling at ropes, reefing, &c.

A swelling, at first small, is seen in the groin, which disappears when the man lies down, and returns when he stands up or coughs; there is little pain, but a feeling of dragging at the lower part of the body. If neglected, the swelling is liable to be nipped by the walls of the passage through which it has come.

The channel of the bowel is then closed, the swelling cannot be pushed back into the belly, and is then said to be strangled. In such a case the swelling in the groin is elastic, and more or less painful to the touch. The patient at first has pain in the bowels, which are obstinately confined; after a short time, he vomits, and eventually brings up excrement, when his condition is, of course, very dangerous.

Treatment.—Give the man from 40 drops to a dram of laudanum, put him in a warm bath at a temperature of 100 degrees Fahr^t, and keep the water at that temperature.

When the patient feels faint from the heat of the bath, the swelling is to be pressed very gently and steadily upwards, always following the direction in which it has come down.

Be careful not to use too much force, as by so doing the bowel may be much injured. The attempt to put it back should not be continued for more than twenty minutes or half an hour.

The patient must now be taken out of the bath, wiped dry, and put to bed. If the above treatment has not succeeded, and snow or ice be handy, a bladder or oil-silk bag filled with either is to be kept for some hours on the swelling, and often, under the constant application of cold, the swelling is so reduced that the bowel is easily pushed back.

All men who are ruptured should be supplied with a truss at the earliest opportunity.

RETENTION OF URINE.

That is, when a man is unable to pass his water. It is caused—

(1) By holding the water too long after a desire to pass it, or after drinking heavily.

(2) By Stricture.

(3) By Clap.

(4) By an injury to the passage, and by falling on or striking the crutch.

(5) By long-continued exposure to wet or cold.

Treatment.—Give the patient 40 or 50 drops of laudanum, place him in a bath at 100 degrees Fahr', and keep it at that temperature for a quarter of an hour. The patient will often pass a little water in the bath, which will give great relief. If, however, these means fail, try to introduce a catheter gently into the bladder.

How to introduce a Catheter.—Make the patient stand up against a bulkhead, and sit down in front of him. Having taken the wire out of the instrument, oil the latter, and hold it like a pen between the fingers of your right hand. The yard of the patient must be held in your left hand, and the instrument gently put into the passage, and pushed steadily on into the bladder. The instrument must be held loosely between the fingers, and *on no account must any force be used.* If any obstacle be met with, overcome it by steady and moderate pressure, *and not by sudden force.* The entrance of the instrument into the bladder is at once shown by a flow of urine. If you do not succeed after a quarter of an hour's trial, leave off for a time. A dose of salts should be given to clear out the bowels, and afterwards another dose of laudanum. If this fail, the warm bath should be repeated, and the stricture will generally yield a little, allowing, at all events, a small quantity of urine to dribble away.

Sometimes, after severe straining, the patient feels that something has given way suddenly, and is immediately relieved. This is a very dangerous sign, for it indicates that the passage has burst behind the stricture, and that the urine has escaped into the neighbouring parts. In a few hours the yard begins to swell, the skin becomes tight and shiny, and the patient complains of a burning pain in the crutch. He will be able to pass water, but the relief is only of a temporary nature.

It is necessary in such a case to push a lancet deeply into the middle of the fork, behind the purse, *taking care to keep exactly in the middle line,* in order to give escape to the urine. Small cuts must also be made on each side of the purse, to let out the water there collected. Keep up the strength of your patient with good food and wine or grog, and see that the wounds are well washed with warm carbolic acid lotion at least three times a day.

DRIBBLING OF URINE

May be caused—

(1) By Piles.

(2) By Stricture.

(3) By a stone in the bladder.

In children it may be caused by worms in the lower part of the bowel.

Treatment.—Little can be done at sea in the way of treatment. If the patient be a lad, and he wets his bed-clothes at night, let him be roused at the end of every watch and made to pass water. In older patients, no satisfactory treatment can be adopted by a non-professional man, except by giving a double dose of the soothing mixture (page 74) now and then at bed-time.

BOILS.

BOILS.—These are very common among sailors, and are generally caused by constant irritation of skin from saltwater—hence the term 'saltwater boils.'

Treatment.—When the boil is beginning to form, rub it with lunar caustic, and, if very painful, put over it lint dipped in a weak mixture of rum and water. Linseed-meal poultices should afterwards be used, and in time the boil will soften, the core come out, and the hole close. You will help the healing by using the basilicon ointment.

If the patient be of full habit, give him a black draught twice a week.

WHITLOW.—Inflammation of the fingers, with great pain and swelling. The pain is deep and throbbing, and the skin red, swollen, and shiny. It is most frequently caused by running a splinter of wood under the nail, or into the finger.

Treatment.—Whitlows should be treated early, for the fingers may be lost by extension of the inflammation to the deep parts.

As soon as the back of the finger or hand is red, swollen, and puffy, make a deep cut lengthways along *the middle* of the finger *in front*, to allow the escape of matter. A poultice must then be applied and changed frequently, but in spite of all care the first bone of the finger will sometimes be killed.

ULCERS.

These are of various kinds.

HEALTHY ULCERS are of a bright red colour, are covered with small red growths, and discharge a thick yellowish matter.

Treatment.—Lint dipped in warm water and kept constantly moist.

INFLAMED ULCERS.—These are very painful; the surrounding parts are hot and red, the discharge is small in quantity, of a dark colour, and has sometimes a foul smell.

Treatment.—The patient must knock off work, and a linseed poultice, or carbolic acid lotion, cold or warm, mixed with laudanum (page 76), must be constantly applied on a rag; the bowels should be opened by a dose of salts.

ULCERS DEPENDING UPON ENLARGED VEINS.—This variety is always found on the legs. The skin near the ulcer is of a purplish brown, and beneath it are seen the swollen knotty veins. The edges of the ulcer are hard and thick, its surface smooth and dead-looking, and there is but little discharge. These ulcers may open one of the enlarged veins and cause serious bleeding. If this occur, let your patient lie down, with his leg raised, and while he is in this position, make steady pressure on the bleeding spot, and keep up the leg and the pressure until the blood ceases to flow.

Dress the ulcer with Goulard lotion, and bandage the affected limb as smoothly and evenly as possible.

PILES.

A feeling of itching, heat, and swelling about the vent, and a straining after stool, as if there were something more to come.

Piles may be inside or outside, bleeding or blind.

Piles within the vent often bleed; but those outside give no trouble, if kept perfectly clean.

The inward piles often come down when the bowels

are moved, especially if the patient has had a hard motion. Sometimes a pile is caught by the muscle which closes the vent, and, if thus caught, cannot get up again after the action of the bowels. If this occur, a bluish swelling is seen protruding from the vent, which is painful, hot, and tender. This swelling should be at once returned, which is easily done by smearing it with olive oil, and pushing it up gently with the forefinger.

Treatment.—The bowels should be kept open by a teaspoonful of sulphur given every morning, and the parts must be carefully washed after every action of the bowels. Cleanliness is very important. If the piles bleed, give an injection of the soothing lotion (page 75).

GUM-BOIL.

The pain is very severe, especially at night. A small cut should be carefully made into the swelling with a lancet, and instant relief will follow the escape of matter.

BLEEDING FROM THE NOSE.

This is nature's remedy for the cure of headache, and should not be interfered with. If, however, it be very severe, cold applied to the nose and to the back of the neck will be all-sufficient, except in very obstinate cases, when the nostrils must be very gently and carefully plugged with lint, rag, or a piece of sponge.

r

Scale of Medicines issued and caused to be published by the Board of Trade in pursuance of the Merchant Shipping Act, 1867.

NOTE.—The column for the use of Druggists is not inserted here.

Names of Medicines, Medicaments, &c.	Proportion for Ships carrying the undermentioned No. of Men and Boys (for 12 months)		
	10 and under	11 to 20 inclusive	21 and upwards
Alum	1 oz.	2 oz.	3 oz.
Balsam of copaiba . . .	4 ,,	8 ,,	12 ,,
Bicarbonate of soda . . .	8 ,,	12 ,,	16 ,,
Black draught . . .	1 pint	2 pints	3 pints
Black wash . . .	1 ,,	2 ,,	2 ,,
*Carbolic acid . . .	½ gal.	1 gal.	2 gals.
Castor oil	1 lb.	2 lbs.	3 lbs.
Cream of tartar . . .	2 oz.	4 oz.	8 oz.
†Condy's crimson fluid . .	½ pint	1 pint	1 pint
Epsom salts . . .	3 lbs.	6 lbs.	12 lbs.
Essence of peppermint . .	—	1 oz.	2 oz.
,, ,, ginger . .	—	1 ,,	2 ,,
Goulard's extract . .	1 oz.	2 ,,	4 ,,
Iodide of potassium . .	—	2 ,,	4 ,,
Laudanum . . .	2 oz.	4 ,,	8 ,,
Linseed meal . . .	—	14 lbs.	28 lbs.
Lunar caustic . . .	¼ oz.	½ oz.	1 oz.
Nitrate of potash . .	2 ,,	4 ,,	8 ,,
Ointment, basilicon . .	3 ,,	6 ,,	10 ,,
Ditto mercurial . .	1 ,,	2 ,,	4 ,,
Ditto simple . .	6 ,,	12 ,,	16 ,,
Olive oil	—	8 ,,	12 ,,
Opodeldoc . . .	8 oz.	6 ,,	10 ,,
Paregoric	4 ,,	6 ,,	8 ,,
Pills, blue . . .	1 doz.	2 doz.	3 doz.
Ditto, cough . . .	2 ,,	4 ,,	6 ,,
Ditto, opium . . .	1 ,,	2 ,,	3 ,,
Ditto, purging . . .	3 ,,	6 ,,	8 ,,
Ditto, mild . . .	3 ,,	6 ,,	8 ,,
Powder, compound rhubarb .	2 oz.	4 oz.	8 oz.
‡ Ditto, diarrhœa . .	1 ,,	2 ,,	3 ,,
Ditto, Dover's . .	1 ,,	2 ,,	3 ,,
Ditto, ipecacuanha . .	1 ,,	2 ,,	3 ,,
‡Quinine	1 ,,	2 ,,	3 ,,
Solution of chloride of zinc . .	4 pints	8 pints	16 pints
Spirits of nitric ether . . .	—	2 oz.	3 oz.
Sulphate of zinc . . .	1 oz.	2 ,,	3 ,,
Sulphur (sublimed) . . .	4 ,,	6 ,,	8 ,,
Tincture of henbane . . .	1 ,,	2 ,,	3 ,,
,, ,, rhubarb . .	4 ,,	10 ,,	12 ,,
Turpentine liniment . . .	2 ,,	4 ,,	6 ,,

antiseptic and deodorising agent for common use.
'fying drinking water when necessary.
he quantity above indicated to be taken to all tropical ports.

Scale of Medical Stores issued and caused to be published by the Board of Trade in pursuance of the Merchant Shipping Act, 1867.

Scales of Medical Stores and Necessaries	Proportion for Ships carrying the undermentioned No. of Men and Boys (for 12 months)		
	10 and under	11 to 20 inclusive	21 and upwards
Adhesive plaster on unbleached calico in tin case . . .	1 yard	2 yards	3 yards
Lint	½ lb.	¾ lb.	1 lb.
Scales and weights . . .	1 set	1 set	1 set
Graduated drop measure . .	—	1	1
Graduated 2-oz. measure . .	1	1	1
6-oz. bottles	½ doz.	½ doz.	1 doz.
Corks for ,, ...	1 ,,	1½ doz.	2 ,,
Scissors	—	1 pair	1 pair
Syringes	2	2	4
Lancet	1	1	1
Abscess ditto . . .	1	1	1
Bandages	—	6	6
Calico	3 yards	4 yards	6 yards
Flannel	2 ,,	3 ,,	6 ,,
Needles, pins, thread, and tape .	—	1 paper	1 paper
Splints, common . . .	1 set	1 set	1 set
Trusses	1	1	1
Enema syringe . . .	1	1	1
Pewter cup	—	1	1
Teaspoon (pewter) . . .	—	1	1
Bougies	1 set	1 set	1 set
Catheter	1	1	1
Bed pan	—	1	1
Arrowroot	2 lbs.	4 lbs.	8 lbs.
Pearl barley . . .	4 ,,	8 ,,	16 ,,
Rice	4 ,,	8 ,,	16 ,,
Corn flour	4 ,,	8 ,,	16 ,,
Sago	4 ,,	8 ,,	16 ,,
Sugar	14 ,,	28 ,,	56 ,,
Soup and bouilli . . .	6 ,,	12 ,,	24 ,,
Boiled mutton . . .	6 ,,	12 ,,	24 ,,
Essence of beef . . .	6 tins (¼ pint)	12 tins	24 tins
Compressed vegetables (mixed) .	4 lbs.	8 lbs.	16 lbs.
Potato (if not in scale of provisions)	14 ,,	28 ,,	56 ,,
Wine (port) . . .	3 bottles	6 bottles	12 bottles
Brandy	2 ,,	4 ,,	6 ,,

DOSES AND DIRECTIONS FOR USE OF MEDICINES.

THE doses of these medicines are calculated for men, so that half the quantity should be in all cases given to children under sixteen years of age, and the names of all *outward* applications are printed in thick black type (as Alum, &c.) to distinguish them from medicines that are to be taken internally.

Alum.—1 dram in a pint of water is a useful gargle for a sore throat.

BALSAM OF COPAIBA.—A good remedy for the clap.   (See Receipt No. 5.)
Dose : half a dram.

BICARBONATE OF SODA.—Useful for indigestion. Forty grains mixed in a glass of water with an ounce of lime or lemon-juice makes a refreshing effervescent drink.   (See Receipt No. 6.)
Dose : 10 to 40 grains.

BLACK DRAUGHT.—The best purgative.
Dose : 1 oz.

Black Wash.—A lotion for chancres.

Carbolic Acid.—To be mixed with water, and used for washing decks, bunks, and all places in which foul smells exist.

A tablespoonful in each bucket of water for washing decks and bunks, and half that quantity for scrubbing clothes or washing the skin, will be quite sufficient. (See also Receipt No. 11.)

According to the scale published by the Board of Trade, the carbolic acid may be either liquid or crystal; but whether liquid or crystal is carried, it must contain in each 100 parts not less than 80 parts of carbolic (or phenic) and cresylic acids and their homologues, and not more than 20 parts of water.

Whatever variety be used, attend to the directions printed on the case or bottle.

CASTOR OIL.—A good and safe purgative.
Dose: 1 oz. to 1½ oz.

CREAM OF TARTAR.—An useful purgative for certain cases, as directed in this book.
Dose: 20 grains to a dram.

Condy's Crimson Fluid.—Two or three drops into each gallon of water wanting purification for drinking purposes.

EPSOM SALTS.—A good purgative when it is necessary to repeat the dose.
Dose: ½ oz. to 1½ oz.

ESSENCE OF PEPPERMINT. — To flavour other medicines.

Dose: 10 to 20 drops.

ESSENCE OF GINGER. (See Receipt No. 6.)

Dose: 5 to 20 drops.

Goulard's Extract.—For external application only. (See Receipt No. 9.)

IODIDE OF POTASSIUM.—To be given only as directed in this book.

Dose: 5 to 8 grains in an ounce of water.

LAUDANUM.—Useful to stop diarrhœa, to ease pain, and to procure sleep. In doses larger than those indicated, it is poisonous.

Dose: 6 to 40 drops.

Linseed Meal.—For Poultices. (See Receipt No. 15.)

Lunar Caustic.—For external application; to be used only as directed in this book. (See Receipt No. 8.)

NITRATE OF POTASH.—Useful in fever mixtures. (See Receipts No. 1 and 2.)

Dose: 15 grains to half a dram.

Ointment (Basilicon).—For sores that will not heal with the use of simple ointment. Spread it sparingly on a rag, as much grease makes dirt, and does more harm than good.

Ointment (Mercurial).—To be used only for crabs, and rubbed in sparingly.

Ointment (Simple).—To be sparingly spread on a rag for sores and blisters. (See also Receipt No. 14.)

Olive Oil.—To smear over piles in aiding their return, and to paint over burns of the face.

Opodeldoc.—For external application only. To be used sparingly. Rubbing it on the skin relieves rheumatic and other pains.

PAREGORIC.—To relieve obstinate coughing in cases of bronchitis and consumption.

Dose: 1 teaspoonful occasionally.

BLUE PILLS.—To be used only as directed in this book.

COUGH PILLS.—One to be taken now and then for a troublesome cough.

OPIUM PILLS.—These pills must be used cautiously.

1 for a dose, to procure sleep.

PURGING PILLS.—One or two to be taken at night to open the bowels.

MILD PURGING PILLS.—One or two to be taken at night, to open the bowels.

COMPOUND RHUBARB POWDER. (See Receipt No. 6.)

Dose: 20 grains to a dram.

DIARRHŒA POWDER.—To stop purging of the bowels.

Dose: 20 grains to a dram.

DOVER'S POWDER.—To procure rest and sweating. To be used only as directed in this book.

Dose: 10 to 12 grains.

IPECACUANHA.—In *acute* dysentery.

Dose: 5 to 15 grains.

QUININE.—This should be measured out carefully in the quantities directed, kept as powder, and each mixed just before drinking in a glass of water. To be used only as directed in this book.

Dose: 2 to 10 grains.

Solution of Chloride of Zinc.—For cleansing and deodorising purposes. To be used according to the directions printed on the bottle.

SPIRITS OF NITRIC ETHER.—(See Receipts No. 2, 4, and 5.)

Dose : 30 drops to a dram.

SULPHATE OF ZINC.—(See Receipt No. 12.)

Dose : half a dram in a glass of water, to cause vomiting; and 2 grains in an ounce of water, as an injection for the clap.

SULPHUR.—To open the bowels gently.—(See also Receipt No. 14.)

Dose : A teaspoonful in a glass of water, or any other fluid.

TINCTURE OF HENBANE.—To be used only as directed in this book. (See Receipt No. 4.)

Dose : 30 drops to a dram.

TINCTURE OF RHUBARB.

Dose : 1 to 2 drams to be given with 15 grains of soda and 10 drops of laudanum, in 2 oz. of water, twice a day, for gripes without much looseness.

Turpentine Liniment.—For external application only. (See Receipt No. 13.)

RECEIPTS.

1.—*Saline Mixture.*

Nitrate of potash . . . 1½ dram
Water . . . . . 6 oz.

2 tablespoonfuls for a dose.

2.—*Fever Mixture.*

Nitrate of potash . . . 1½ dram
Spirits of nitric ether . . 3 drams
Add water to . . . . 6 oz.

2 tablespoonfuls for a dose.

3.—*Diarrhœa Mixture.*

Diarrhœa powder . . . 2 drams
Laudanum . . . . 1 dram
Add water to . . . . 6 oz.

2 tablespoonfuls for a dose.

4.—*Soothing Mixture.*

Tincture of henbane . . . 3 drams
Spirits of nitric ether . . 3 drams
Add water to . . . . 6 oz.

2 tablespoonfuls for a dose.

5.—*Clap Mixture.*

(This must be well shaken.)

Balsam of copaiba . . .	3 drams
Spirits of nitric ether . .	1 dram
Add water to	6 oz.

2 tablespoonfuls for a dose.

6.—*Stomachic Mixture.*

Compound rhubarb powder .	2 drams
Bicarbonate of soda . . .	3 drams
Essence of ginger . . .	1 dram
Add water to	6 oz.

2 tablespoonfuls for a dose.

7.—**Alum Gargle.**

Alum	1 dram
Warm water	6 oz.

8.—**Caustic Lotion.**

Lunar caustic	1 dram
Rain water	6 oz.

9.—**Goulard Lotion.**

Goulard's extract . . .	1 dram
Add *rain* water to . . .	6 oz.

10.—**Soothing Lotion.**

Goulard's extract . . .	1½ dram
Laudanum	2 drams
Add *rain* water to . . .	6 oz.

11.—Carbolic Acid Lotion.

Carbolic acid   .   .   .   . $\frac{1}{2}$ oz.
Add *rain* water to   .   .   .   6 oz.

12.—Clap Injection.

Sulphate of zinc   .   .   .   12 grains
Rain water   .   .   .   .   6 oz.

13.—Turpentine Fomentation.

Soak a large square of rag in the turpentine liniment, and put it on the skin; wring out in hot water
any old square of flannel or woollen stuff at hand,
put this over the turpentine rag, and over both a
layer of cloth or any convenient clothing to keep in
the heat. Let the fomentation remain on at least
twenty minutes.

14.—Sulphur Ointment.

Mix thoroughly 2 oz. of sulphur with 8 oz. of lard,
simple ointment, or any other grease that is procur-
able.

15.—Linseed Poultice.

Use boiling water. Add linseed meal to the water
in very small quantities, and mix well, so that the
poultice may not be lumpy; spread it quickly and
smoothly with a cold wet spoon on linen rag, and put
it on the part as hot as it can be borne.

ACT OF PARLIAMENT.

CERTAIN SECTIONS OF THE MERCHANT SHIPPING ACT, 1867.

SECTION 4.

(2) The owners of every ship navigating between the United Kingdom and any place out of the same shall provide and cause to be kept on board such ship a supply of medicines and medical stores in accordance with the scale appropriate to the said ship, and also a copy of the said book or of one of the said books containing instructions.

(3) No lime or lemon juice shall be deemed fit and proper to be taken on board any such ship, for the use of the crew or passengers thereof, unless the same has been obtained from a bonded warehouse for and to be shipped as stores; and no lime or lemon juice shall be so obtained or delivered from any warehouse as aforesaid unless the same is shown, by a certificate under the hand of an inspector appointed by the Board of Trade, to be proper for use on board ship, such certificate to be given upon inspection of a sample after deposit of the said lime or lemon juice in the warehouse; nor unless the same contains

fifteen per centum of proper and palatable proof spirits, to be approved by such inspector, or by the proper officer of customs, and to be added before or immediately after the inspection thereof; nor unless the same is packed in such bottles, at such time and in such manner, and is labelled in such manner as the Commissioners of Customs may direct; provided that when any such lime or lemon juice is deposited in any bonded warehouse, and has been approved as aforesaid by the said inspector, the said spirits, or so much of the said spirits as is necessary to make up fifteen per centum, may be added in such warehouse, without payment of any duty thereon; and when any spirit has been added to any lime or lemon juice, and the same has been labelled as aforesaid, it shall be deposited in the warehouse for delivery as ship's stores only, upon such terms and subject to such regulations of the Commissioners of Customs as are applicable to the delivery of ship's stores from the warehouse.

(4) The master or owner of every such foreign-going ship (except those bound to European ports or to ports in the Mediterranean Sea, and also except such ships or classes of ships bound to ports on the eastern coast of America north of the thirty-fifth degree of north latitude, and to any islands or places in the Atlantic Ocean north of the same limit, as the Board of Trade may from time to time exempt from this enactment) shall provide and cause to be kept

on board such ship a sufficient quantity of lime or lemon juice from the warehouse duly labelled as aforesaid, such labels to remain intact until twenty-four hours at least after such ship shall have left her port of departure on her foreign voyage, or a sufficient quantity of such other anti-scorbutics, if any, of such quality, and composed of such materials, and packed and kept in such manner, as Her Majesty by order in council may from time to time direct.

(5) *The master of every such ship as last aforesaid shall serve or cause to be served out the lime or lemon juice with sugar (such sugar to be in addition to any sugar required by the articles), or other such anti-scorbutics as aforesaid, to the crew so soon as they have been at sea for ten days, and during the remainder of the voyage, except during such time as they are in harbour and are there supplied with fresh provisions; the lime or lemon juice and sugar to be served out daily at the rate of an ounce each per day to each member of the crew, and to be mixed with a due proportion of water before being served out, or the other anti-scorbutics, if any, at such times and in such quantities as Her Majesty by order in council may from time to time direct.*

(6) If at any time, when such lime or lemon juice or anti-scorbutics is or are so served out as aforesaid, any seaman or apprentice refuses or neglects to take the same, such neglect or refusal shall be entered in

the official log-book in the manner provided by the two hundred and eighty-first section of the principal Act, and shall be signed by the master, and by the mate or some other of the crew, and also by the surgeon or medical practitioner on board, if any.

And if in any such ship as aforesaid such medicines, medical stores, book of instructions, lime or lemon juice, sugar, or anti-scorbutics as are hereinbefore required are not provided, packed, and kept on board as hereinbefore required, the owner or master shall be deemed to be in fault, and shall for each default incur a penalty not exceeding twenty pounds, unless he can prove that the non-compliance with the above provisions, or any of them, was not caused through any inattention, neglect, or wilful default on his part; and if the lime or lemon juice and sugar or other anti-scorbutics are not served out in the case and manner hereinbefore directed, or if entry is not made in the official log in the case and manner hereinbefore required, the master shall be deemed to be in fault, and shall for each default incur a penalty not exceeding five pounds, unless he can prove that the non-compliance with the above provisions, or any of them, did not arise through any neglect, omission, or wilful default on his part; and if in any case it is proved that some person other than the master or owner is in default in any case under this section, then such other person shall be liable to a penalty not exceeding twenty pounds.

SECTION 5.

Any person who manufactures, sells, or keeps, or offers for sale, any such medicines or medical stores as aforesaid which are of bad quality shall. for each such offence incur a penalty not exceeding twenty pounds.

SECTION 6.

In any British possession out of the United Kingdom, the governor, or officer administering the government for the time being, shall, subject to the laws of such possession, have power to make regulations concerning the supply within such possession of lime or lemon juice and anti-scorbutics for the use of ships; and any lime or lemon juice or anti-scorbutics duly supplied in accordance with any such regulations shall be deemed to be fit and proper for the use of ships.

SECTION 7.

Whenever it is shown that any seaman or apprentice who is ill has, through the neglect of the master or owner, not been provided with proper food and water according to his agreement, or with such accommodation, medicines, medical stores, or anti-scorbutics as are required by the principal Act or by this Act, then, unless it can be shown that the illness has been produced by other causes, the owner or master shall be liable to pay all expenses properly and necessarily incurred by reason of such illness (not exceeding in

G

the whole three months' wages), either by such seaman himself, or by Her Majesty's government, or any officer of Her Majesty's government, or by any parochial or other local authority on his behalf, and such expenses may be recovered in the same way as if they were wages duly earned: Provided that this enactment shall not operate so as to affect any further liability of any such owner or master for such neglect, or any remedy which any seaman already possesses.

Section 8.

Where a seaman is by reason of illness incapable of performing his duty, and it is proved that such illness has been caused by his own wilful act or default, he shall not be entitled to wages for the time during which he is by reason of such illness incapable of performing his duty.

Section 10.

The following rules shall be observed with respect to the medical inspection of seamen; that is to say,

(1) At any port where there is a Local Marine Board, the Local Marine Board, and at other ports in the United Kingdom, the Board of Trade may appoint a medical inspector of seamen.

(2) Such medical inspector of seamen shall, on application by the owner or master of any ship, examine any seaman applying for employment in such ship, and shall give to the superintendent of

the Mercantile Marine Office a report under his hand stating whether such seaman is in a fit state for duty at sea, and a copy of such report shall be given to the master or owner of the ship.

(3) The master or owner applying for such inspection shall pay to the superintendent such fees as the Board of Trade direct, and such fees shall be paid into and form part of the Mercantile Marine Fund.

(4) The said medical inspectors shall be remunerated for their services as the Board of Trade may direct, and such remuneration shall be paid out of the Mercantile Marine Fund.

(5) In British possessions out of the United Kingdom, the governor or other officer administering the government for the time being shall have the power of appointing medical inspectors of seamen, of charging fees for inspections, when applied for, and of determining the remuneration to be paid to such inspectors.

FORM OF CERTIFICATE OF BIRTH.

BIRTH OF A CHILD AT SEA ON BOARD

Date of Birth	Name	Sex	Name and Surname of Father	Name and Maiden Surname of Mother	Rank or Profession of Father	Signature of Master of Ship

LIST OF CAUSES OF DEATH.

The preceding list of causes of death is appended for use in connection with the certificate. It is compiled from the list of diseases used by the Registrar-General of Births and Deaths for England and Wales, and is believed to contain the names of all mortal maladies likely to occur at sea.

A strict adherence to this brief list will very greatly assist the efforts of the Registrar-General of Seamen in obtaining from the official log-books accurate returns of mortality at sea.

FORM OF CERTIFICATE OF DEATH.

DEATH AT SEA ON BOARD

Date of Death	Name	Sex	Age	Rank or Profession	Cause of Death	Signature of Master of Ship

INDEX.

LONDON: PRINTED BY
SPOTTISWOODE AND CO., NEW-STREET SQUARE
AND PARLIAMENT STREET

DISINFECTION BY OXYGEN.

CONDY'S PATENT FLUID,

Which is entirely DEVOID OF SMELL and ABSOLUTELY INOFFENSIVE, is the best, the safest, the cheapest, and only agreeable disinfectant for all ordinary disinfecting purposes, such as

**PURIFYING INFECTED BEDDING AND LINEN,
ARRESTING CONTAGIOUS DISEASES,
CLEANSING BILGES, HOLDS, BUNKS, CABINS, PANTRIES, &c.,
AND EXTIRPATING BAD ODOURS WHEREVER THEY EXIST,**

as well as for many others, for which it alone can be used;
as, for instance,

REMOVING TAINT AND SMELL FROM OFFENSIVE WATER AND DAMAGED OR UNSOUND MEAT.

CONDY'S FLUID is the only known Agent by means of which Vessels which have been loaded with Sugar or Guano can be thoroughly purified so as to be fit for carrying Tea and such-like delicate cargoes. It is also of great use for removing the smell left by Carbolic Acid.

N.B.—For the purification of Water, be particular to use only
CONDY'S FLUID (**CRIMSON**).

To make down, for general use, Condy's Fluid, which is a concentrated preparation, add one teaspoonful to a pint of water, or one wineglassful to a bucket. One half-pint bottle makes ten bucketfuls for use.

PRICES.

In Bottles (Green), 1s. and 2s., or in Bulk, 5s. per Gallon; (Crimson) stronger and purer, 1s., 2s., and 4s:, or in Bulk, 10s. per Gallon. Bottles, 8d. per Gallon in bulk.
Costing, when diluted, from One Farthing to One Halfpenny per Gallon.

A good commission allowed to Captains and Officers of Ships on orders sent or influenced by them.
Condy's Fluid can be had from the Proprietors, with Labels and Directions for Use in most foreign languages.
Commanding Officers are respectfully requested to report to the Board of Trade (Marine Department) the results obtained by them from the use of Condy's Fluid on b. ard ship, and their opinion of its general utility.

⁎⁎ *Purchasers must be careful to look for the above Trade Mark—without which the article cannot be genuine.*

H. BOLLMANN CONDY, Patentee, Battersea, London.
For Testimonials, see over.

FROM MEDICAL AND OTHER REPORTS IN FAVOUR OF CONDY'S FLUID.

(OUT OF MANY HUNDREDS.)

Conclusions drawn by Dr. Bérenger-Féraud from the Experiments made by him at Havre on Disinfectants on board the Imperial yacht 'Jérome-Napoléon.'

'1. Wood charcoal is radically inefficient and inapplicable.

'2. Chlorine and chloride of lime are hurtful as well as inefficient.

'3. Carbolic acid is of no use, and has an insupportable odour.

'4. Protosulphate of iron may for the present be preferred; it is sufficiently active to be of considerable use, and very low in price.

'5. Permanganate of potash (Condy's Fluid) is infinitely superior to all the preceding substances, and is destined to put them all into the shade. The purifying action of this substance is so remarkable that its success in the disinfection of putrid matters of very kind may safely be assumed. It effectually destroys the foul odours arising from suppuration and from putrefying and fæcal matters. I have derived the greatest advantage from its use for many other sanitary purposes besides those just mentioned.'—On the Comparative Action of various Disinfecting Agents, with reference to the Purification of Ships' Bilges, by Dr. Bérenger-Féraud, Surgeon to the Imperial yacht 'Jérome-Napoléon.'—*Medical Press and Circular*, June 10, 1868.

'Liverpool, June 17, 1858.

'I can testify to the complete destruction, by Condy's Fluid, of the smell of guano in the "Salem," and I am the owner of that ship.   J. G. STUART.'

'23 Park Street, Bristol, August 1, 1860.

'SIR,—I have used your Fluid during the last two-and-a-half years in many ways, and am perfectly satisfied of its value. It possesses advantages over other disinfectants with which I am acquainted by rendering the air cool, refreshing, and entirely free from smell, and without injuring clothes and furniture. In recovering, and preventing taint in meat, it is particularly successful. The meat is plunged into the diluted solution, taken out and hung up, and, when cooked, it is entirely free of all unpleasant taste.   I am, Sir, yours truly,

'To Mr. Condy.   AUG. TALBOT, M.D.'

'Condy's Fluid is the best if not the only purifier of water for drinking. As much as will tinge the water a delicate pink suffices to destroy all organic impurities; and for restoring a healthful principle to the air, pieces of linen rag or flannel, steeped in Condy's Fluid, diluted with about ten times its bulk of water, should be hung upon strings about a house as linen is hung upon clothes lines to dry. An important part has been played by this disinfectant in the work of purifying the London Hospital.'— ON CHOLERA DISINFECTION, *Daily Telegraph*, August 4, 1866.

'Most practical physicians have seen the immediate action of Condy's Fluid in disinfecting the sick-room; and it has often occurred to myself to limit malignant forms of disease to the room occupied by the sufferer, by nailing a sheet, saturated with that Fluid diluted, over the doorway leading to other parts of the house.'—*Report on the Measures taken against the Cholera in the City of London in 1866*, by Dr. W. S. SAUNDERS, Superintending Medical Adviser to the Board of Guardians, p. 10.

'31 Theadneedle Street, London, Nov. 1, 1867.

'SIR,—I have much pleasure in communicating to you an extract from a letter received this day from the Chairman of the Anglo-Greek Committee, Athens, which is as follows:—"Condy's Fluid has been found to be of great service in the Military Hospital, in which a contagious disease had appeared. The chief surgeon speaks in high terms of approbation of the valuable effects of this disinfectant in purifying the atmosphere of the hospital, and arresting the progress of gangrene among the wounded Cretan invalids.'

'On behalf of the Anglo-Greek Committee,—Yours obediently,

'H. B. Condy, Esq.   STAUROS DILBEROGLUE.'

'Bexley Heath, Kent, February, 15, 1867.

'SIR,—After an experience of several years on board ship and dispensary practice, I can bear testimony to the efficacy of your Fluid. Having caused it to be used in ships' bilges, it was reported to me to be the best deodorizer ever tried. In the close cabin of a vessel, when from heavy weather the ports were obliged to be tightly screwed in, I found it totally destroy all fetor in a most offensive surgical case. The same happy results were obtained by me from its use in the filthy, over-crowded rooms of the poor, in an atmosphere reeking with the emanations from the excreta of cholera patients, during the late epidemic in Liverpool. As a local application to foul and indolent ulcers, it not only totally destroys all smell but produces a healthy action in the sore. I consider that no ship or dispensary ought to be without adequate supplies of Condy's Fluid.   Yours faithfully,

'H. B. Condy, Esq.   N. W. BARRINGTON, A.B., M.R.C.S., M.D.'

The Royal Alfred Belvedere Institution
FOR DISABLED AND WORN-OUT MERCHANT SEAMEN.

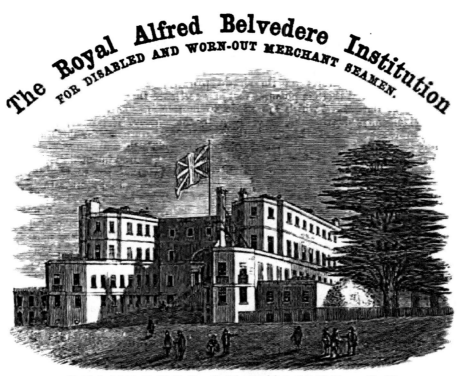

BELVEDERE-ON-THAMES, S.E.
(*Supported by Voluntary Contributions.*)

Patron—H. R. H. CAPTAIN THE DUKE OF EDINBURGH, R.N., K.G., K.T.

This is a Home for our old *Merchant Sailors*, Officers and Men, who are above 60 years of age, and have served 21 years in the Mercantile Marine of the United Kingdom, and who have *no friends living to take care of them*. Those old Seamen of the same standing who have wives or relatives with whom to reside, will receive help from the Institution, so far as the funds will admit of it, so that there will be no need of the workhouse should they be unable to support themselves.

The Institution was opened on January 1st, 1867, when a number of *friendless* old Sailors were elected into the House, and a proportionate number, *having relative ties*, were pensioned out, receiving 8d. a day, or £12 a year. Elections have taken and will take place from time to time, as circumstances shall admit, funds alone being wanted to increase the number to 500 at Belvedere-on-Thames, and to erect similar Institutions at other large seaports.

Masters, Mates, and Seamen will establish a *claim* to the benefits of the Institution by becoming Sub- scribers, as follows, viz.:—

Masters and First Mates, an Annual Subscription of 10s. each; Seamen, an Annual Subscription of 5s. each; other Mates may pay which Subscription they please—ranking accordingly—for which a Ticket will be given.

It is hoped that you who subscribe may never want; but if you do, it will be a proud satisfaction, when participating in its benefits, that in your young days you lent a generous hand to support it.

Your Subscriptions will be received by your Captain, or, when on shore, by the Honorary Agents of the Shipwrecked Mariners' Society throughout the kingdom (who also act as Honorary Agents for Belvedere Institution), and by the Secretary, Hibernia Chambers, London Bridge, by Post-Office Order, Stamps, or otherwise.

NOTICE.

For Masters, Mates, and Seamen who have no relatives living, and who would wish to leave their Property to THE ROYAL ALFRED BELVEDERE INSTITUTION, the following ' **Form of Will** ' is suggested :—

' I, *Master, Mate, or Seaman (as the case may be)* on board the Ship
give and bequeath to the ROYAL ALFRED BELVEDERE INSTITUTION, FOR WORN-OUT AND DISABLED MERCHANT SEAMEN, *all my PERSONAL ESTATE, and all wages that may be due to me at the time of my death.*
Signature of
this   day of   18.
To be signed by two persons as witnesses, and lodged with the Captain or other responsible person.

COUNTERFEITS.

'ENVY will merit as its shade pursue,' says a philosophic poet; and there is no surer test of excellence than the number and variety of the efforts which are made to imitate it. This reflection, we conceive, may afford some consolation to the *Messrs. Rowlands*, whose admirable requisites for the toilet—their Matchless *Macassar* for the Hair, *Kalydor* for the Complexion, and *Odonto* for the Teeth and Gums—are, from their merit and reputation, the constant objects of fraudulent imitation both at home and abroad. There is, however, this difference, that, while the French legal authorities denounce such practices, and prohibit their continuance, even though the sufferer by such fraud be a foreigner, and not a native of France, our own laws are not sufficiently stringent or precise in this particular for the prevention of crime; and thus unprincipled and needy adventurers are found, who, by imitating the articles, and even the advertisements, pass off the vile trash as 'Real *Macassar Oil*,' 'True *Kalydor*,' &c., regardless alike of their own character or reputation, and of the injury inflicted by their vile compounds on the unsuspecting public.

One safeguard of course remains; the purchaser has only to inspect the signature, and to ascertain that it is that of Messrs. ROWLAND & SONS, as no others are genuine. Being productions of art and manufacture, they are far from cumbrous, and consequently easy of transit; while their finding a ready sale, and maintaining an unalterable value, make them at once an available and certain source of fair remunerating profit to the

MERCHANT, CAPTAIN, AND SHIPPER.

SHIPWRECKED FISHERMEN & MARINERS' ROYAL BENEVOLENT SOCIETY.

SHORT TITLE—

SHIPWRECKED MARINERS' SOCIETY

(Incorporated by Act of Parliament, and supported by voluntary contributions).

Patron—HER MOST GRACIOUS MAJESTY THE QUEEN.

President—His Grace the Duke of MARLBOROUGH, D.C.L.

Chairman of Committee.
Captain Hon. FRANCIS MAUDE, R.N.

Deputy Chairman of Committee
WILLIAM STUART, Esq.

Secretary—FRANCIS LEAN, Esq., R.N.
Second Secretary—Capt. W. H. SYMONS, R.N.

Travelling Secretaries,
W. C. PRINCE, JAMES BANCKS, N. CUMMING, and LINDON SAUNDERS, Esqs.

Collector—Mr. A. F. STRETTELL.

The Society, by means of the Secretary and about 900 Honorary Agents, distributed round the coast, minister immediate relief to shipwrecked men of all nations landed on our shores, clothing and sending them to their homes; or, if Foreigners, to their nearest Consuls. The widows and orphans of the drowned fishermen and mariners are liberally relieved. (James i. 2, 7.)

As the number of wrecks increase with the number of ships, so as to more than average 10 per diem, the Committee are obliged to pressingly appeal to the benevolent Public for pecuniary help to meet the continual wants of the poor castaways. (Acts xxviii. 2.) They succour in this trying hour on an average annually between 11,000 and 12,000 persons.

Donations and Annual Subscriptions will be thankfully received in Stamps, Cheques, or Post Office Orders, by Messrs. Williams, Deacon, and Co., Birchin Lane, City, Bankers to the Society; by all the London and County Bankers; by the several Metropolitan Army and Navy Agents; by the Honorary Agents throughout the kingdom; by the Travelling Secretaries, Collector, and at the Office of the Society,

HIBERNIA CHAMBERS, LONDON BRIDGE, S.E.

The Society also publish a Quarterly Marine Magazine, 'THE SHIPWRECKED MARINER,' price 6d. May be had of GEORGE MORRISH, 24 Warwick Lane, Paternoster Row, or through any bookseller.

THE BEST REMEDY FOR INDIGESTION!!

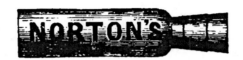

CAMOMILE PILLS

Are confidently recommended as a simple but CERTAIN REMEDY FOR INDIGESTION, which is the cause of nearly all the diseases to which we are subject, being a Medicine so uniformly grateful and beneficial that it is with justice called the 'Natural Strengthener of the Human Stomach.' NORTON'S PILLS act as a powerful tonic and gentle aperient; are mild in their operation; safe under any circumstances; and thousands of persons can now bear testimony to the benefits to be derived from their use.

Sold in Bottles at 1s. 1½d., 2s. 9d. and 11s. each, in every Town in the Kingdom.

CAUTION !—Be sure to ask for 'NORTON'S PILLS,' and do not be persuaded to purchase the various imitations.

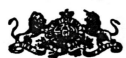

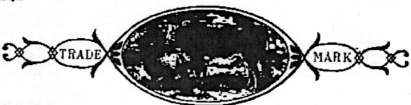

CPSIA information can be obtained at www.ICGtesting.com
Printed in the USA
BVOW05s1530160115

383672BV00016B/252/P